Histological Classification
of
Bone and Joint Tumors of Domestic Animals

Histological Classification *of* Bone and Joint Tumors of Domestic Animals

Compiled and Reviewed by:
M. V. Slayter, T. R. Boosinger, R. R. Pool,
K. Dämmrich, W. Misdorp, and S. Larsen

Second Series
Volume I

With 53 Figures

Published by the Armed Forces Institute of Pathology
in cooperation with the American Registry of Pathology and
The World Health Organization Collaborating Center
for Comparative Oncology
Washington, D.C.
1994

Available from
American Registry of Pathology
Armed Forces Institute of Pathology
Washington, D.C. 20306-6000
ISBN: 1-881041-12-3
1994

The Participants of Volume I

- *DR. T. R. BOOSINGER*
  Department of Pathobiology, College of Veterinary Medicine, Auburn University, Auburn, Alabama, U.S.A.

- *DR. K. DÄMMRICH*
  Institute for Veterinary Pathology, Freie Universität Berlin, Germany.

- *DR. S. LARSEN*
  Department of Pharmacology and Pathobiology, the Royal Veterinary and Agricultural University, Frederiksberg, Denmark.

- *DR. W. MISDORP*
  Department of Pathology, Faculty of Veterinary Medicine, University of Utrecht, The Netherlands.

- *DR. R. R. POOL*
  Department of Veterinary Pathology, School of Veterinary Medicine, University of California, Davis, California, U.S.A.

- *DR. M. V. SLAYTER*
  Department of Veterinary Pathology and WHO Collaborating Center for Comparative Oncology, Armed Forces Institute of Pathology, Washington, D.C., U.S.A.

Acknowledgements

Materials for this volume were from the archives of the Armed Forces Institute of Pathology (AFIP); The Ohio State University, College of Veterinary Medicine; the University of California, Davis, School of Veterinary Medicine; and the WHO Collaborating Center for Comparative Oncology. Camera-ready layout was performed by Ms. Fran Card; color separation by Mr. Kenneth Stringfellow; and color photography was done by Ms. Robin-Anne V. Ferris, all of the AFIP.

Preface

In 1974 and 1976, the World Health Organization published the International Histological Classification of Tumors of Domestic Animals.* Since that time there has been a substantial increase in the body of knowledge concerning animal neoplasms and extensive refinement in classification schemes. The original series, published in twenty chapters, each dealing with a major organ system, is clearly in need of revision. This monograph on the classification of orthopedic tumors in domestic animals represents the first of the second series of tumor classifications. The second series will again be organ-based and will be published as individual monographs. Their publication represents the results of a cooperative program sponsored by the Armed Forces Institute of Pathology (AFIP), the American Registry of Pathology (ARP), and the World Health Organization (WHO). It is our intent that this series, like the first, serves to cross geographic and academic boundaries and establishes an international consensus pertaining to the nomenclature of domestic animal neoplasms.

We undertake this task as part of our responsibility as the WHO Collaborating Center for Comparative Oncology. Those who would like to participate in the production of a second series monograph should contact the Department of Veterinary Pathology, Armed Forces Institute of Pathology.

* WHO. International Histological Classification of Tumors of Domestic Animals. *Bull. World Health Organ.*, Vol. 50, No. 1–2, 1974; and Vol. 53, No. 2–3, 1976.

Contents

INTRODUCTION

This is a classification of primary tumors and tumor-like lesions of bones and joints of domestic animals and is a revision of the first International Histological Classification of Tumors of Domestic Animals, published in the *Bulletin of the World Health Organization* in 1976. Like the first series, this scheme is based primarily on histological criteria. Tumors of bone have been divided into two groups, benign tumors and malignant tumors, based on cellular features. The benign and malignant groups are subdivided based on the type of cellular matrix made by the cells and on the anatomic location of the tumor in a given bone (central vs. peripheral). In sarcomas with mixed cell types the tumor is named based on the malignant potential of the predominate cell type.

The accurate diagnosis of bone and joint tumors requires adequate clinical and radiographic evaluations of the lesion as well as histology. Without this information the significance of the microscopic findings in a small biopsy specimen may be misinterpreted. A definitive diagnosis may require multiple biopsies.

The clinical history should include the duration, size, and location of the lesion plus the effect of the lesion on locomotion. A minimum of two radiographic views will help establish the size, shape, and precise anatomic location of the tumor. The selection of a biopsy site should be judged by radiography, and the biopsy should be large enough to include both the center and the margin of the tumor. Necropsy specimens usually provide the most valuable diagnostic information, especially if they are processed and evaluated as oversized whole-mount specimens.

Primary bone tumors are observed most frequently in dogs and cats and are rare in other domestic animals. Benign tumors of bone are very uncommon but, when observed, are reported most frequently in cattle and horses. Sarcomas of bone are primarily a disease of dogs and cats. Eighty percent of primary malignant bone tumors in dogs, and fifty percent in cats, are osteosarcoma. Chondrosarcomas are the second most common histologic type in dogs. The incidence of sarcomas in dogs, especially osteosarcoma, is highest in giant breed dogs and boxer dogs. In dogs osteosarcomas develop three to four times more often in the appendicular skeleton than in the axial skeleton.

Histological Classification of Bone and Joint Tumors of Domestic Animals

I. BENIGN TUMORS

A. Osteoma
B. Ossifying fibroma
C. Myxoma of the jaw
D. Osteochondroma
E. Feline osteochondromatosis
F. Chondroma
G. Hemangioma

II. MALIGNANT TUMORS

A. Central
   1. Osteosarcoma
      a. poorly differentiated
      b. osteoblastic
         - nonproductive
         - productive
      c. chondroblastic
      d. fibroblastic
      e. telangiectatic
      f. giant cell type
   2. Chondrosarcoma
   3. Fibrosarcoma
   4. Hemangiosarcoma
   5. Giant cell tumor of bone
   6. Multilobular tumor of bone

B. Peripheral
   1. Periosteal chondrosarcoma
   2. Periosteal fibrosarcoma
   3. Maxillary fibrosarcoma (dogs)
   4. Periosteal osteosarcoma
   5. Parosteal osteosarcoma

C. Joint tumors
   1. Synovial sarcoma
D. Miscellaneous tumors
   1. Liposarcoma
   2. Malignant mesenchymoma
   3. Others
E. Tumors of bone marrow
   1. Myeloma
   2. Malignant lymphoma

III. TUMOR-LIKE LESIONS

A. Fibrous dysplasia
B. Solitary bone cyst
C. Juxtacortical bone cyst
D. Epidermoid cyst of the phalanx
E. Myositis ossificans
F. Villonodular synovitis

Definitions and Explanatory Notes

I. BENIGN TUMORS

A. Osteoma *(Figs. 1, 2)*

An infrequently occurring benign, usually solitary, tumor found mostly on the head and composed of essentially normal, mature well-differentiated bone.

Grossly, the tumor has a smooth contour, protrudes from a surface, and blends with the underlying resident bone. Histologically, the tumor is composed of dense coalescing spicules and trabeculae of bone lined by the usual compliment of osteoblasts and osteoclasts. The intertrabecular connective tissue is composed of spindle cells and becomes increasingly sparse as the tumor becomes more compact and sclerotic. Due to the rarity of cases, a species predilection seems unlikely. Malignant progression has not been reported.

B. Ossifying fibroma *(Fig. 3)*

A rare, usually solitary, slow-growing expansile tumor that is morphologically a fibroma that contains metaplastic bone.

Synonyms include fibrous osteoma and osteofibroma. In animals, it occurs in the jaw and is composed of spindle cells that undergo transformation to osteoblasts as they line spicules of bone. The osseous component is usually woven spicular bone centrally and lamellar bone peripherally. Unlike the osteoma, it replaces normal underlying tissue. This tumor should be differentiated from fibrous dysplasia.

C. Myxoma of the jaw *(Figs. 4, 5)*

An uncommon tumor of stellate cells and gelatinous matrix which, when involving bone, has a predilection for the jaws of large animals.

The microscopic appearance is that of embryonal tissue. The matrix is composed of proteoglycans, loose reticulum, and collagen fibers. The tumor may be incompletely lobulated and is usually unencapsulated. There should be no foci of further differentiation such as osseous or chondroid areas. Malignant varieties do occur and are identified initially by their more rapidly invasive nature. The benign examples are also invasive but very slow growing.

D. Osteochondroma *(Fig. 6)*
E. Feline osteochondromatosis *(Figs. 7–10)*

Usually multicentric, cartilage-capped, partially ossified protuberances that resemble an epiphyseal plate that is rotated 90 degrees to the long axis of the bone.

Many theories exist as to their origin. Histologically the cartilage cells mimic the same zones of development found in a normal epiphysis, even to the point that the lesions will mature as the animal matures and will stop growing at the time of growth plate closure. In dogs and horses, the lesions are of clinical significance only when mechanical interference is created. However, malignant transformation has occurred in long-standing lesions of older animals. Because of the more serious consequences of lesions in cats, it is important to note that osteochondromas in dogs and horses never occur on bones of intramembranous origin, such as in the skull. In cats, however, the tumors arise after skeletal maturity, have a random distribution including the skull, demonstrate progressive growth like a tumor, and have viral particles resembling feline leukemia virus (FELV) and feline sarcoma virus (FSV) in the proliferating cells located at the surface of the lesion. Malignant transformation (osteosarcoma) of these benign lesions can occur in cats, as can the appearance of new lesions, imparting a grave prognosis to all feline cases. The term "osteochondromatosis" is especially applicable in the cat because of the unique features described above.

F. Chondroma *(Figs. 11, 12)*

A rare benign tumor of mostly mature cartilage that is usually encapsulated, slowly expanding, smooth to nodular, and lacks all the malignant features of chondrosarcoma, such as multinucleated cells, cellular atypia, and invasion.

These tumors usually arise from flat bones and ribs rather than long bones and can be solitary or, rarely, multiple. While areas of gelatinous myxoid-like material may suggest less advanced differentiation, they are not a sign of malignancy. Areas with mineralization, fibrous tissue, and bone tissue may be produced. In some cases there may be more fibrous stroma present than is found in normal hyaline cartilage. Erroneously, many other proliferations that contain cartilage, such as mixed mammary tumors, synovial chondroma, osteochondroma, etc., have been lumped into this category.

G. Hemangioma of bone *(Fig. 13)*

A primary bone tumor with large cavernous, blood-filled, endothelial-lined spaces with all histologic features being well-differentiated.

Although normally considered in the category of soft tissue tumors, this lesion can arise as a primary tumor in bone and has histologic features that parallel the soft tissue counterpart. Malignant transformation does not occur; however, a periosteal reaction may ensue. Resident bone tissue may be destroyed by tumor expansion. The main feature distinguishing hemangioma from telangiectatic osteosarcoma is the lack of an endothelial lining in the latter.

II. MALIGNANT TUMORS

Primary sarcomas of bone can be divided into two categories, central and peripheral, with the former being the largest by far in terms of incidence and concern. The largest and most heterogeneous group is that of osteosarcoma, a primary malignant mesenchymal tumor that makes osteoid and bone. Because of the varied histologic appearances of bone tumors, especially malignant examples, the goal of this section is to aid in the recognition of the different types.

Bone tumors present certain difficult features because they

must be considered within the context of the whole tumor and the whole animal in order to be accurately and consistently assessed. Frequently, soft tissue tumors reveal their biological nature in small biopsy specimens. The true nature of bone tumors, however, often requires multiple biopsies, radiographs, and clinical follow-up. For this reason, radiographs and gross presentations are emphasized in this text. Although tumor types are usually named for the matrix they produce, it is the cells that impart the significant biological features to the tumor. Throughout the discussion of bone tumors, a pivotal point in the determination of malignancy is the recognition of cell variation in (1) size, (2) staining, and (3) shape. This becomes increasingly important when the pathologist is presented with limited material, such as a punch biopsy, and no radiographs. A usual dilemma stems from the fact that bone tumors are named according to the matrix they produce and may contain multiple cell types and matrices. Furthermore, secondary or metastatic tumors may assume a different appearance from the primary, with different component proportions. The biological behavior is often not apparent, unless biopsies or radiographs indicate the damage imparted to the surrounding tissue or the bone from which the tumor arose.

Generally, disease effects its changes by employing and accentuating normal mechanisms. The growth of a bone tumor induces change in normal bone by stimulating clast and blast activity, not by direct effect alone. A sclerotic rim around a circumscribed lesion is an adaptation to allow transfer of forces around the space-occupying mass. It is usually found with slow-growing masses (tumors, cysts, etc.). If the lesion is inflammatory, such as an abscess, the outer margins of the rim will not be sharp but fading into the surrounding tissue. A circumscribed lesion with no sclerotic rim is an indication that the rate of bone loss exceeds the rate of bone response and containment of the lesion. Tumor masses that grow by expansion rather than infiltration create a "punched-out" appearance. Localized lesions with an ill-defined margin have a local infiltrative nature.

A moth-eaten appearance consists of multiple lytic lesions that arise separately and may coalesce. This pattern usually starts on the endosteal surface and implies malignancy of moderate aggressiveness or inflammation. In permeative-type cortical destruction, there is accelerated remodeling by cutting cones due to stimulated osteoclastic activity. The latter activity is non-specific and may be due to neoplastic or nonneoplastic mechanisms. The most common error is to misclassify reactive bone as malignant growth. The hallmark of reactive osseous tissue is orderliness of size and proportions regarding cells and trabeculae (Fig. 14).

It bears mentioning that the fastest rate of tumor growth through cancellous bone produces little radiographic change. It displaces the soft tissue of the marrow and fills the spaces between trabeculae, producing an invisible tumor margin.

Secondary (metastatic) tumors in the skeleton of the dog and cat are of diagnostic importance since their clinical and radiological appearance may simulate osteosarcoma or other malignant bone tumors. Secondary tumors can involve bone either by direct extension or by hematogenous metastasis. Blood-borne metastases preferably localize, often in a multiple fashion, in the ribs, vertebrae, and long bones. The metastatic tumors are frequently of epithelial origin, such as mammary gland, lungs, or prostate.

A. Central

1. Osteosarcoma *(Figs. 15–26)*

A primary malignant tumor of mesenchymal tissue that gives rise to a variety of patterns, but always includes the production of bone by malignant osteoblasts.

Most osteosarcomas originate in the medullary cavity of the metaphysis and invade the overlying cortex. As with many malignant mesenchymal tumors, the ability to invade and infiltrate between normal or preexisting structures is usually the primary histologic clue that reveals the biologic behavior of the tumor and its subsequent diagnosis and prognosis (Fig. 15).

Histologically, there may be wide variation within a given individual osteosarcoma as well as between individual cases. The tumor contains broad sheets of somewhat polyhedral cells that also may be round to spindle and give rise to osteoid in varying amounts. The cells may vaguely resemble epithelial cells by having ample cytoplasm and sometimes forming a crude organoid pattern. Pleomorphism and atypia of nuclei and cytoplasm, hyperchromatic chromatin, and bizarre mitoses are the primary individual cytologic criteria for determining malignancy. Evidence of invasiveness both radiologically and histologically should not be overlooked as important criteria of malignancy and may become extremely important in well-differentiated tumors. In fact, a low-magnification view to evaluate the pattern and behavior of a given bone tumor many times offers more information than close scrutiny of individual cells. Scattered multinucleated giant cells are not an uncommon occurrence in osteosarcoma and do not serve to automatically classify a tumor as osteoclastoma. Arriving at a subclassification depends more on recognizing significant variations in the predominant matrix (osteoblastic, chondroblastic, fibroblastic) produced by the tumor rather than by cytologic details.

Bone reacts to the presence of a primary tumor in a manner that is similar to that caused by other destructive agents such as metastatic tumor and infection. The proliferative bony responses formed by tissues within the bone as well as by a reactive periosteum on the surface must be recognized as a reactive response and not interpreted as tumor tissue. Practice and experience cannot be supplanted in this case.

In dogs, osteosarcoma is usually a middle-age disease and has a slightly higher incidence in males. In cats, a wider age range is affected. Generally, most osteosarcomas of dogs produce metastatic disease within six months of clinical onset. However, while some cats with osteosarcoma will develop early metastatic disease, many are euthanized because of locally aggressive behavior of long-standing bone lesions that fail to produce metastatic disease even after several months. In cats, osteosarcoma is more likely to contain large foci of cartilage.

The following classification scheme for osteosarcoma is currently accepted for use by most veterinary pathologists:

a. Poorly differentiated (Fig. 16)
b. Osteoblastic (Fig. 17)
   - Nonproductive (Fig. 18)
   - Productive (Fig. 19)
c. Chondroblastic (Fig. 20)
d. Fibroblastic (Fig. 21)
e. Telangiectatic (Figs. 22–25)
f. Giant cell type (Fig. 26)

Variations in cellular appearance could be the manifestation of the differentiation potential known to exist in mesenchymal tissue, or metaplastic expression, or some other unexplained phenomenon. The whole topic of metaplasia and/or modulation of mesodermal tissues has been controversial since the second half of the 19th century. The unraveling of that puzzle is outside the boundaries of this publication.

The term osteoblastic should not be confused with osteoblastoma, which is a clearly recognized benign entity in humans, containing a number of other required features for identification, not simply osteoblasts alone.

The concept that malignant osseous neoplasms may also contain malignant chrondroblastic or fibroblastic elements is thought-provoking in terms of prognosis. In humans, some believe such histologic features impart a better prognosis. Others do not and speak cautiously in regarding any feature as an indicator of good prognosis with osteosarcoma. Indeed, various animal studies conducted by veterinary pathologists have resulted in similar conflicting opinions about prognostic correlation with histology. There are also those who believe that the microenvironment of an osteosarcoma may dictate the direction of mesenchymal differentiation. This is based on several facts, including the concept that the radiographic nature of an osteosarcoma may change with time. Nevertheless, we illustrate here a variety of appearances for the sake of diagnostic recognition.

Telangiectatic osteosarcoma is an aggressive tumor that destroys preexisting bone and forms blood-filled cysts lined by tumor cells rather than endothelium. Generally, the production of osteoid is less common than in other types of osteosarcoma. The tumor metastasizes easily, produces secondary lesions similar to the primary, and is highly fatal. It is distinguished most easily from hemangiosarcoma by the production of osteoid, the presence of osteoblasts, and lack of endothelium lining the blood-filled cysts.

2. Chondrosarcoma *(Figs. 27–31)*

A primary malignant tumor arising de novo *in bone or superimposed on a previously benign chondroid tumor. It produces chondroid and fibrillar matrix, but never osteoid.*

Bone matrix can be produced in chondrosarcoma and usually arises through some reactive or metaplastic mechanism. Chondrosarcoma can arise from the medullary cavity (central) or periosteum (peripheral), the medullary origin being more common. Chondrosarcomas occur more commonly on flat bones of large breed dogs but are capable of arising in other breeds and other locations. It is the most frequently found bone tumor in sheep. Compared to osteosarcomas, chondrosarcomas metastasize less frequently and at a longer interval after onset of clinical signs. Radiographically, they have what has generally been called a snowflake or popcorn appearance.

3. Fibrosarcoma *(Figs. 32, 33)*

A tumor that arises from stromal elements within the marrow cavity and produces moderately spindle cell patterns typical of soft tissue fibrosarcomas with varying amounts of collagen. This tumor produces no bone or cartilage.

Radiographically, these tumors show evidence of slow bone destruction and cannot be distinguished from many other tumors in the early stages without biopsy.

4. Hemangiosarcoma *(Figs. 34–36)*

A malignant bone neoplasm that arises from blood vascular endothelium in similar fashion to the soft tissue variety.

As implied in the definition, the tumor resembles the counterpart in soft tissue. Vascular channels are present supported by varying amounts of collagenous stroma. The primary differential diagnosis is telangiectatic osteosarcoma because of (1) blood-filled spaces, and (2) the stroma of hemangiosarcoma may become hyalinized to the point of resembling osteoid. Reactive tissue is usually minimal, which should be taken into account if a pathologic fracture is suspected.

5. Giant cell tumor of bone *(Figs. 37, 38)*

A well-vascularized tumor of both mononuclear and mutinucleated cells, the nuclei of which are very similar.

This particular nomenclature is frequently applied incorrectly to osteosarcoma of the giant cell variant. Primary giant cell tumor of animals, according to ultrastructural and histochemical evidence, is derived from primitive bone marrow stromal cells and shares many properties with osteoclasts. In fact, osteoclastoma was and sometimes still is an accepted synonym. In differentiating a primary giant cell tumor from a giant cell variant of osteosarcoma, the former is usually more vascular and contains areas of mononuclear and multinuclear cells, and the similarity of nuclei in both mononucleated and multinucleated cells is most helpful. In osteosarcoma, the mononuclear cells have darker, angular nuclei or some other distinguishing shape clearly different from the multinucleate cells. Giant cell tumors produce little or no osteoid and have a distinct radiologic appearance of expanded, thin cortical bone in what has been called a "soap bubble" appearance.

6. Multilobular tumor of bone *(Figs. 39–42)*

A tumor of multilobular appearance formed by islands containing cartilage and / or bone of varying differentiation separated by intervening septa of spindle cells.

This tumor occurs mostly in dogs but has been found in cats and horses. Its usual location is the skull and rarely the rib. It can be locally aggressive and has been known to undergo malignant transformation (osteosarcoma and chondrosarcoma) and metastasize. This tumor has been compared histologically to the human juvenile aponeurotic fibroma; however, this condition in humans does not occur on the head. In the dog, it was originally called chondroma rodens by Jacobson. From that terminology has evolved the designation "multilobular tumor of bone," to avoid confusion brought on by other names and to not discount the potential for benignancy or malignancy.

Malignancy is usually heralded by overgrowth of one of the elements, increased mitotic activity, loss of orderly architecture and differentiation, and invasion of adjacent tissue.

B. Peripheral

Osteosarcoma, chondrosarcoma, and fibrosarcoma may also arise from the periosteum. These are considered as a separate group because they generally represent slower growing, less malignant entities compared to central sarcomas on the basis of complete case information. With regard to any of the peripheral tumors, there is a high risk of inaccurate diagnosis if the examination is restricted to histological appearance only. These entities constitute excellent examples of the necessity for radiographs and clinical history when classifying any bone neoplasm.

1. Periosteal chondrosarcoma *(Figs. 43–45)*

A malignant cartilaginous tumor than arises de novo *from the periosteum.*

This tumor does not arise from the progression or degeneration of any other tumor that may have chondroid elements. Two patterns exist that are distinctively different. The first contains cytologic features of low- to intermediate-grade malignancy with variable lobulation and resembles central chondrosarcoma. The second pattern lacks lobulation, has less anaplasia, and frequently contains nonneoplastic bone formed through endochondral ossification.

2. Periosteal fibrosarcoma

A malignant tumor that originates from the periosteum and is composed of well-differentiated fibroblasts with abundant collagen and very little atypia or pleomorphism.

The malignant designation is based more, although not exclusively, on biological behavior rather than histology. With time, the underlying bone destruction can be massive.

3. Maxillary fibrosarcoma *(Figs. 46, 47)*

In the dog it is considered as a distinct entity due to the response to radiation hyperthermia therapy.

Histologically, these tumors are less cellular, lack the expected interweaving pattern of other fibrosarcomas, and have a topographical distinction. Fibrosarcomas of the maxilla and of other parts of the head can be differentiated from similar tumors of the oral cavity only in the early stages.

4. Periosteal osteosarcoma *(Figs. 48, 49)*

An osteosarcoma arising from periosteum.

All aforementioned statements concerning cellular morphology of central osteosarcoma apply in this case as well. The behavior of periosteal osteosarcomas is generally less aggressive than that of central osteosarcomas. Invasion of the underlying cortex is commonplace and is a contrasting feature in distinguishing this tumor from parosteal osteosarcoma.

5. Parosteal osteosarcoma

A peripheral osteosarcoma with the potential for possessing fibrous, osseous, and chondroid elements, most of which look more reactive than neoplastic, but are not without minimal features of malignancy such as atypia and pleomorphism.

Parosteal osteosarcoma is sometimes the center of confusion because it is malignant but yet well-differentiated. Like the periosteal tumors, these are slow growing and generally innocuous in comparison to central sarcomas. Radiographically, the underlying cortex maintains its integrity for a relatively long time.

C. Joint Tumors

1. Synovial sarcoma *(Figs. 50–52)*

An uncommon malignant tumor of joints arising from synovioblastic mesenchyme forming firm, tan-colored tissue with indistinct lobules.

In dogs, the most frequent sites include the stifle, elbow, shoulder, antebrachial-carpal, talocrural, and hip joints. The fleshy lobules of tumor tissue that fill the joint may contain focal areas of hemorrhage, necrosis, and in some cases cystic spaces containing mucinous fluid. Histologically, these tumors frequently contain a variable diphasic mixture of spindle-shaped cells forming the fibroblastic component and a synovioblastic component that tends to form more epithelioid-type cells. These cells have hyperchromatic cytoplasm, a slightly eccentric nucleus, and an ovoid, angular, or fusiform shape. They may be arranged in large sheets, in packets, or short cords. The epithelioid cells can sometimes be found lining clefts and tubular cavities. The mitotic index is highly variable. Some synovial sarcomas may contain multinucleated giant cells, but this is not a consistent nor a predominant feature of these tumors. Some synovial tumors may be monophasic and may resemble fibrosarcoma or metastatic carcinoma.

D. Miscellaneous Tumors

1. Liposarcoma

A malignant tumor, like its soft tissue counterpart, characterized by lipoblastic differentiation, as shown by the presence of atypical lipoblasts.

This rare tumor has been reported to occur in the metaphyses of young dogs.

2. Malignant mesenchymoma

A very rare malignant tumor characterized by the presence of multiple types of differentiations (e.g. osteosarcomatous and liposarcomatous).

All examples should have a fibrosarcoma-like pattern and two other independent sarcoma cell types.

3. Others

This includes such rare lesions as myxosarcoma.

E. Tumors of Bone Marrow

1. Myeloma

A malignant tumor, usually showing multiple discrete or diffuse osteolytic involvement, that is characterized by neoplastic plasma cells that show various degrees of immaturity, including atypical multinucleated forms.

The lesions may sometimes be associated with the presence of abnormal proteins in the blood and urine. The vertebrae, pelvis, ribs, and long bones are the most common sites. Lesions are usually found in other organs as well. Myeloma is not rare in the dog, but is infrequent in the cat, pig, and horse.

2. Malignant lymphoma

Primary lymphoma of bone is reported to occur in the metaphyses of long bones of dogs and cats. More often bone marrow is involved as a part of a wide-spread multicentric lymphoma in cattle, dogs, and cats.

Note: These tumors will be covered in more detail in the volume pertaining to hematopoietic tumors.

III. TUMOR-LIKE LESIONS

This category is included for differential purposes to depict examples of nonneoplastic changes that are frequently confused with tumors of bone.

A. Fibrous dysplasia *(Fig. 53)*

A benign condition characterized by whorling loose fibrous connective tissue and spicules of woven bone that lack lining osteoblasts.

This entity is included as a tumor-like lesion due to the necessity of distinguishing it from ossifying fibroma or, less frequently, osteoma. Fibrous dysplasia is an uncommon finding in a variety of species and can be seen in juvenile animals. For this reason, some place it in the category of developmental lesions. This condition can occur in a solitary or multicentric fashion. It usually occurs as a smooth, expanding mass that replaces normal bone structure, has a thin outer shell of bone formed by the periosteum, and has a gritty texture when cut with a knife. Histologically, it contains thin, curved trabeculae of woven bone embedded in a loose fibrous connective tissue stroma. The trabeculae are poorly formed, have no lining osteoblasts, and are sometimes referred to as "naked" spicules. In more mature lesions the woven bone in the spicules is partially or completely replaced by lamellar bone tissue.

B. Solitary bone cyst

A unicameral cavity filled with clear or sanguineous fluid and lined by a membrane of variable thickness of loose connective tissue with scattered osteoclastic cells.

Bands of fibrin-like material of hyalinized or calcified connective tissue are commonly present in the wall. These cysts occur in the long bones of young dogs. The rare aneurysmal variant is characterized by blood-filled spaces separated by septa containing bone trabeculae and osteoclasts. Polyostotic bone cysts are known to occur in Doberman pinscher dogs.

C. Juxtacortical bone cyst

A cystic, often multilocular, lesion made up of fibrous tissue with extensive myxoid change situated in the subchondral bone adjacent to a joint.

These lesions occur particularly in the phalanx of young horses.

D. Epidermoid cyst of the phalanx

An expanding cyst lined by keratinizing squamous epithelium in dogs.

This rare lesion has to be differentiated from the more frequent squamous cell carcinoma in the digit that may infiltrate the phalanx.

E. Myositis ossificans

A reactive lesion located in soft tissues adjacent to bone. The lesion is characterized by proliferation of bone-forming connective tissue.

Cartilage may also be present. This benign lesion can be distinguished from malignant periosteal tumors by its zonal arrangement, in which metaplastic bone forms at the periphery of the lesion. This lesion has been reported to occur in the dog, cat, and pig.

F. Villonodular synovitis

A diffuse nodular inflammatory lesion of joints and tendon sheaths that is characterized by overgrowth of synovial cells, some of which contain fine granules of hemosiderin.

There is often an admixture of macrophages and lymphocytes. Although this lesion can cause erosion of bone, it is considered proliferative rather than neoplastic in nature. The lesion is reported to occur in dogs and goats. A special variant is the villonodular synovitis of the equine metacarpophalangeal joint.

References

1. Beresford WA. *Chondroid Bone, Secondary Cartilage, and Metaplasia.* Baltimore-Munich: Urban & Scharzenberg, 1981.

2. Dahlin, DC. Osteosarcoma, In: *Bone tumors.* 2nd ed. Springfield, Ill: Charles C Thomas; 1967:156-175.

3. Madewell JE, Ragsdale BD, Sweet DE. Radiologic and pathologic analysis of solitary bone lesions. Part I: Internal margins. *Radiol Clin North Am.* 1981;19:715-748.

4. Misdorp W, van der Heul RO. Tumours of bones and joints. *Bull World Health Organ.* 1976;53:265-282.

5. Palmer N. Bones and Joints. In: Jubb KVF, Kennedy PC, Palmer N, eds. *Pathology of Domestic Animals.* 4th ed. San Diego, Calif: Academic Press Inc.; 1993;1:1-181.

6. Pool RR. Tumors of Bone and Cartilage. In: JE Moulton, ed. *Tumors in Domestic Animals.* Berkeley, Calif: University of California Press; 1990:207-213.

7. Ragsdale BD, Madewell JE, Sweet DE. Radiologic and pathologic analysis of solitary bone lesions. Part II: Periosteal reactions. *Radiol Clin North Am.* 1981;19:749-783.

8. Revell PA. Bone tumors and tumor-like conditions. In: *Pathology of Bone.* Berlin, Heidelberg: Springer-Verlag; 1986: chap 11.

9. Sweet DE, Madewell JE, Ragsdale BD. Radiologic and pathologic analysis of solitary bone lesions. Part III: Matrix patterns. *Radiol Clin North Am.* 1981;19:785-814.

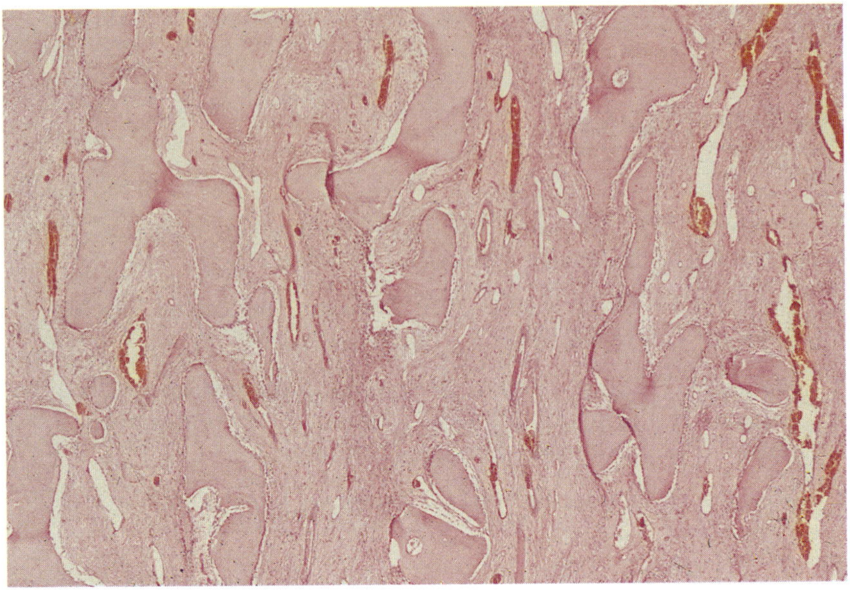

Fig. 1 - Osteoma, horse. This benign tumor is composed of mature, dense coalescing trabeculae lined by osteoblasts and osteoclasts in normal proportions.

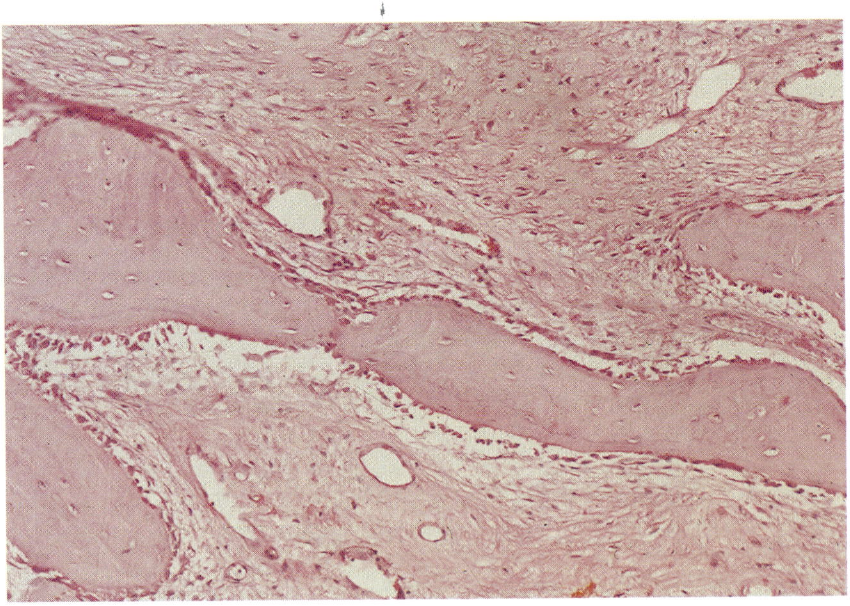

Fig. 2 - Osteoma, horse. Higher magnification of Figure 1. The intervening connective tissue is composed of normal spindle cells and collagen.

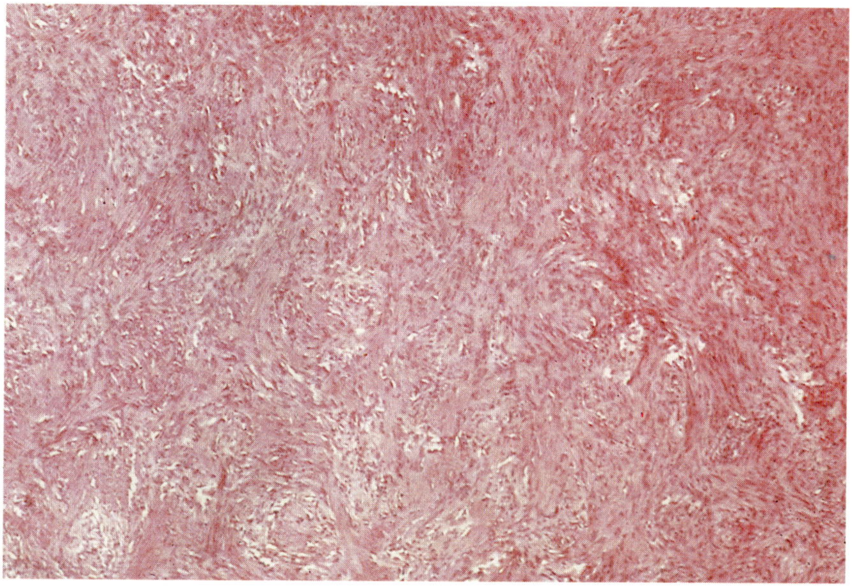

Fig. 3 - Ossifying fibroma. The tumor is composed of benign fibroblasts that blend with productive osteoblasts forming bone.

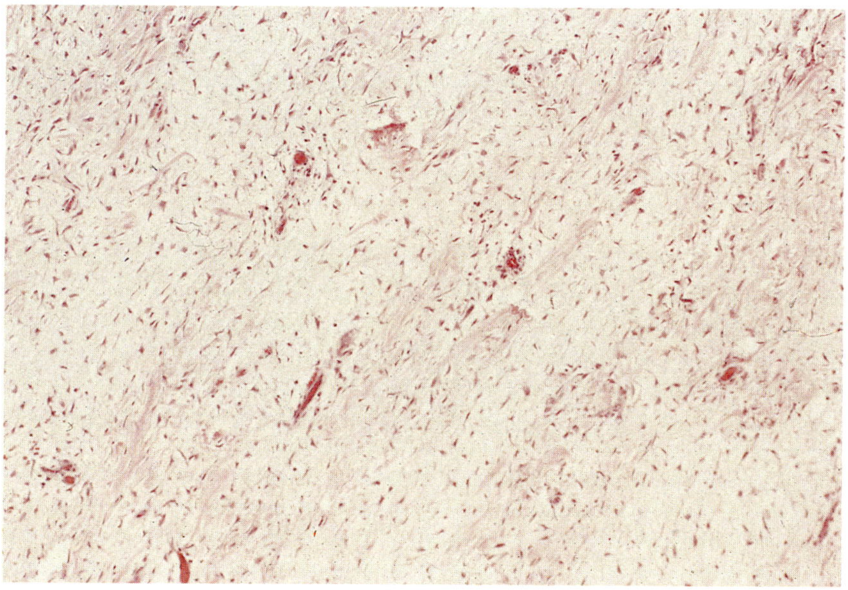

Fig. 4 - Myxoma, jaw, immature horse. The tumor is composed of stellate cells in a gelatinous matrix.

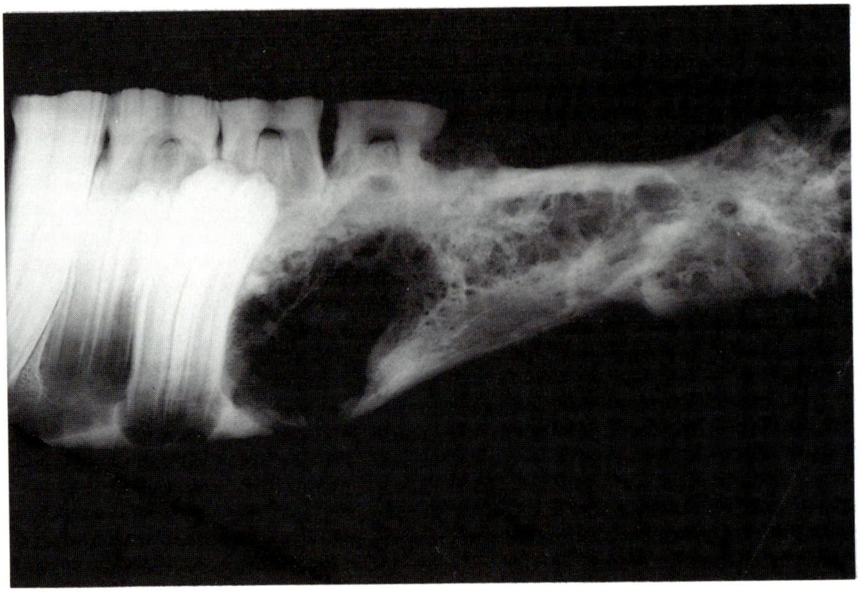

Fig. 5 - Myxoma. Specimen radiograph. Same animal as Figure 4. Destructive lesion of rostral part of mandible is present.

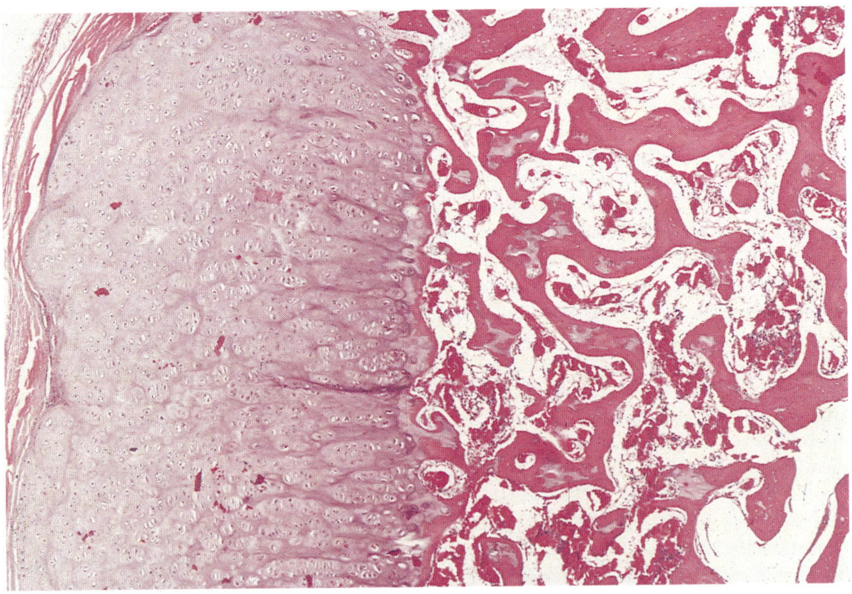

Fig. 6 - Osteochondroma, rib, horse. An epiphyseal-like arrangement of cartilage cap typifies the actively growing stage of this lesion in horses and dogs.

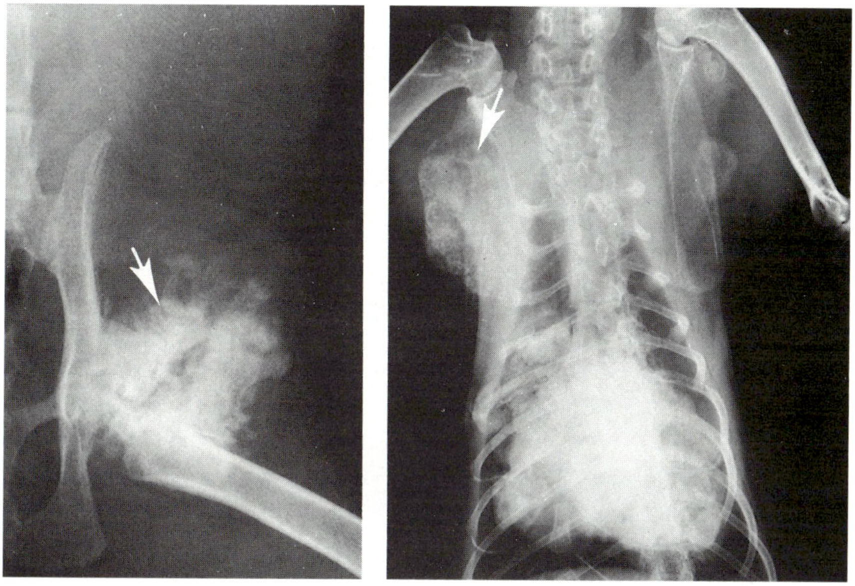

Fig. 7 - Osteochondromatosis, cat. Radiographs showing multiple tumor sites (arrows).

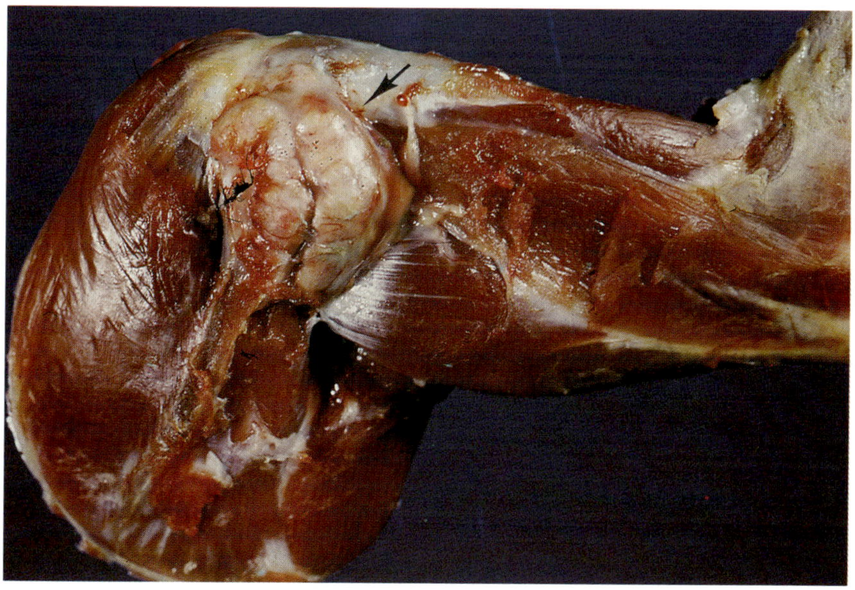

Fig. 8 - Osteochondromatosis (arrow), scapula, cat. Gross photo.

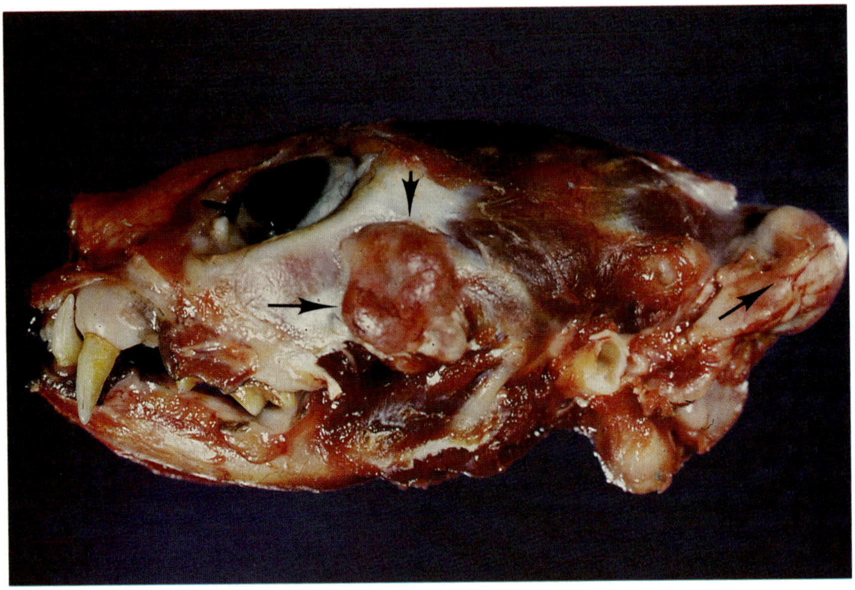

Fig. 9 - Osteochondromatosis, skull, cat. Gross photo showing masses (arrows) on zygomatic process and occipital bone.

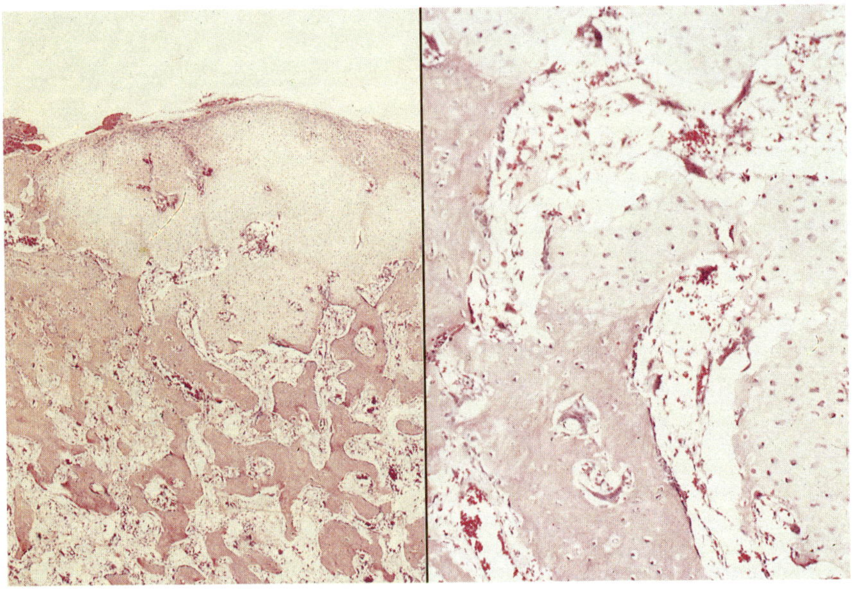

Fig. 10 - Osteochondromatosis, cat. Histologic appearance showing irregularity of the cartilage and haphazard arrangement of chondrocytes giving rise to cancellous bone.

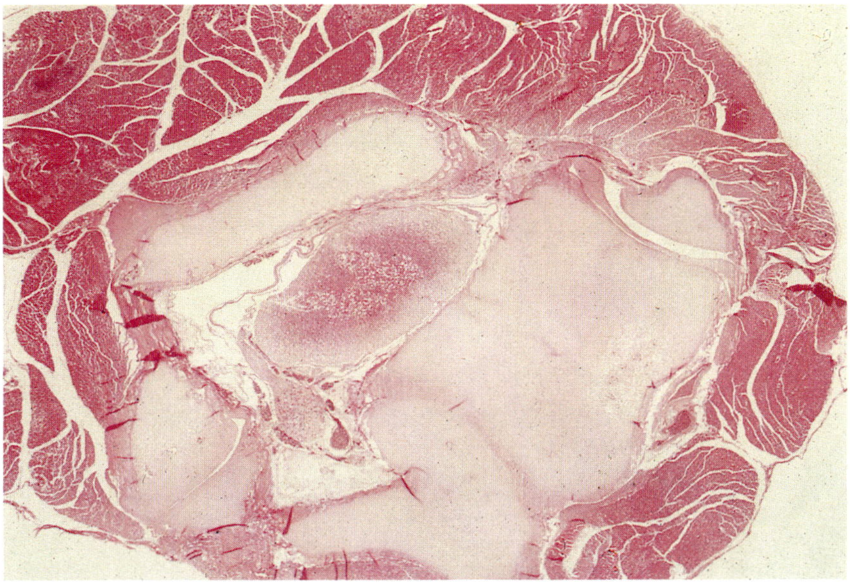

Fig. 11 - Chondroma. The tumor contains well-demarcated islands of mature cartilage.

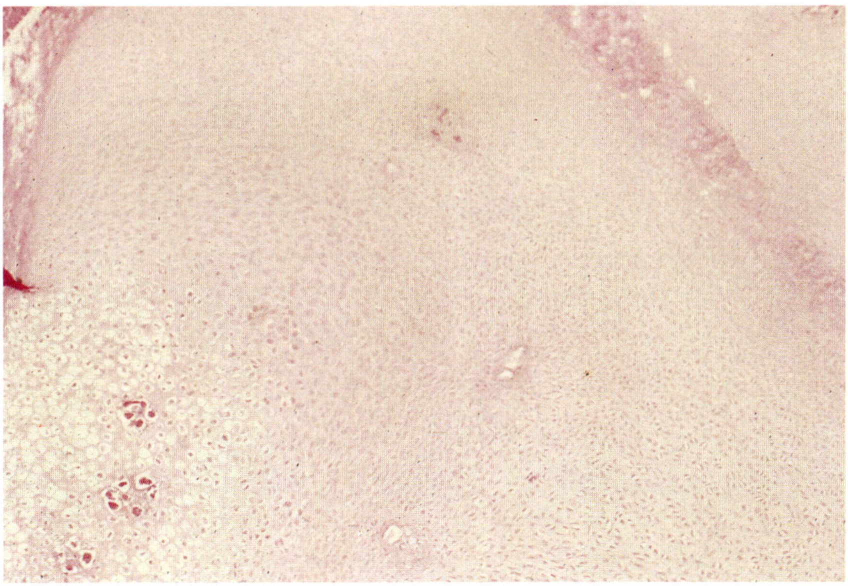

Fig. 12 - Chondroma, hyoid bone, cow. Chondrocytes in lacunae show no atypical features.

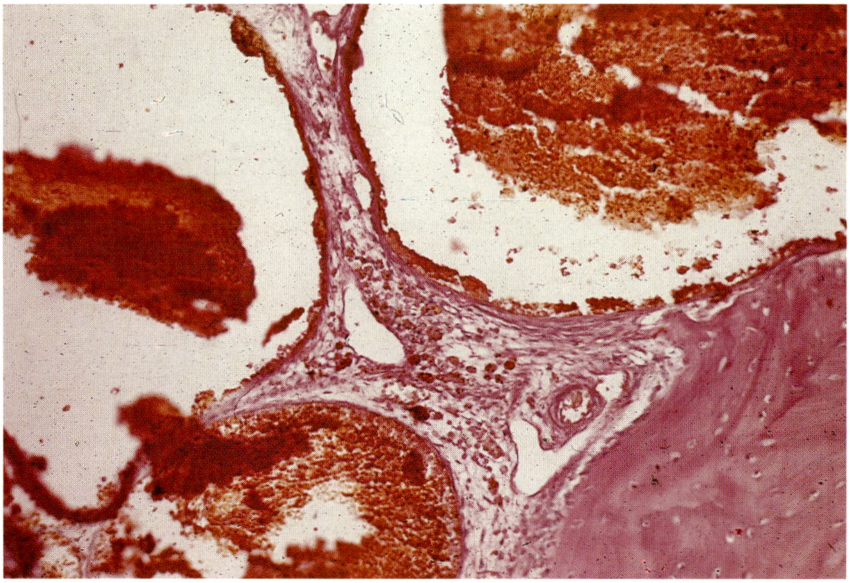

Fig. 13 - Hemangioma, lumbar vertebra, dog. As in its soft tissue counterpart, the blood-filled spaces are lined by well-differentiated endothelium.

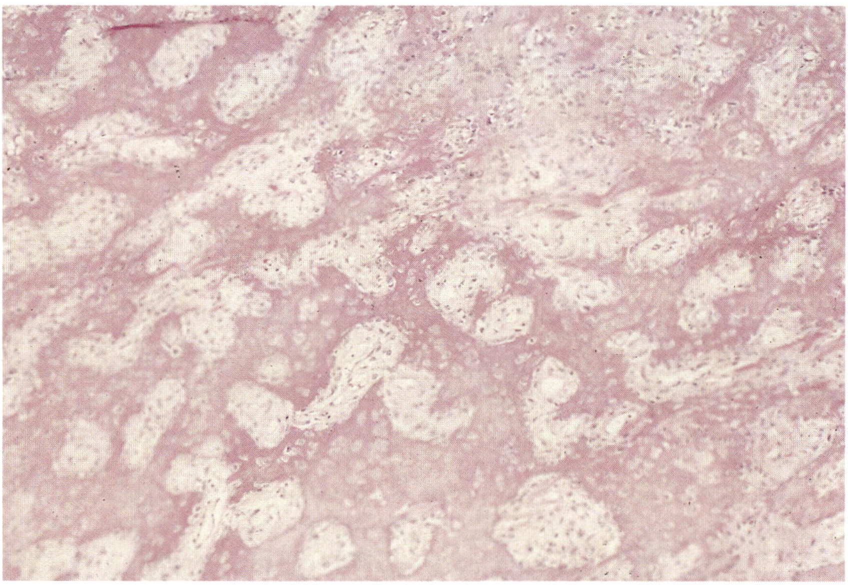

Fig. 14 - Reactive bone. The interconnected, fairly uniform-sized trabeculae lined by normal osteoblasts distinguish this from an osteosarcoma.

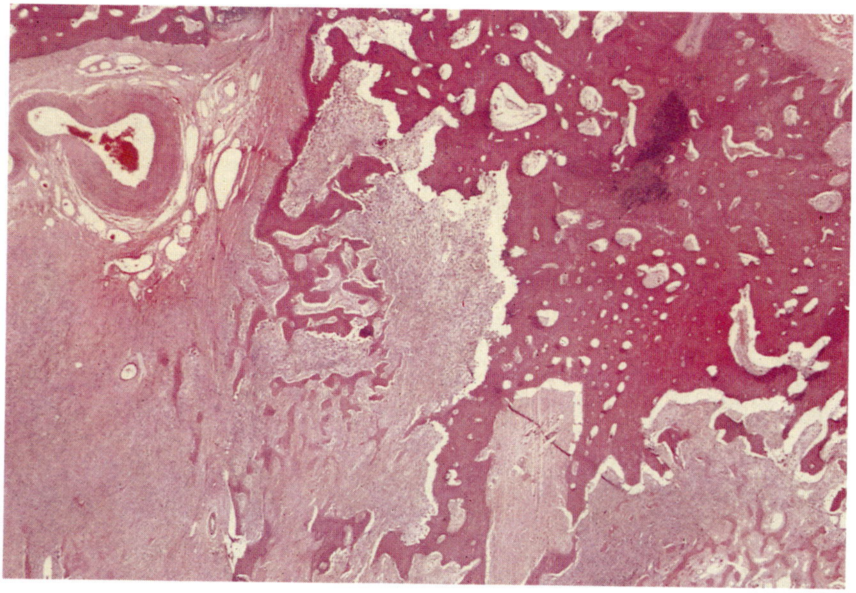

Fig. 15 - Advancing edge of an osteosarcoma. Invasion of tumor into pre-existing bone.

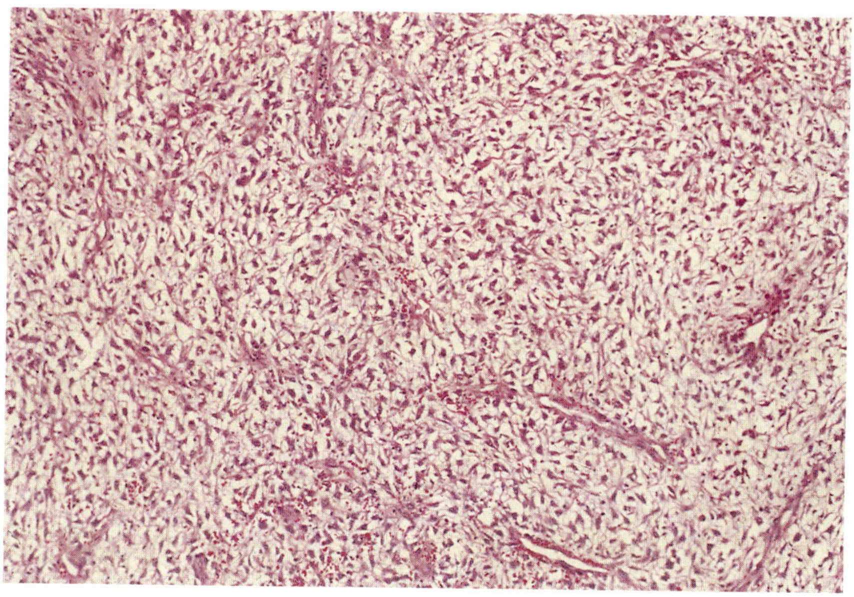

Fig. 16 - Osteosarcoma, poorly differentiated. The cells resemble primitive mesenchyme.

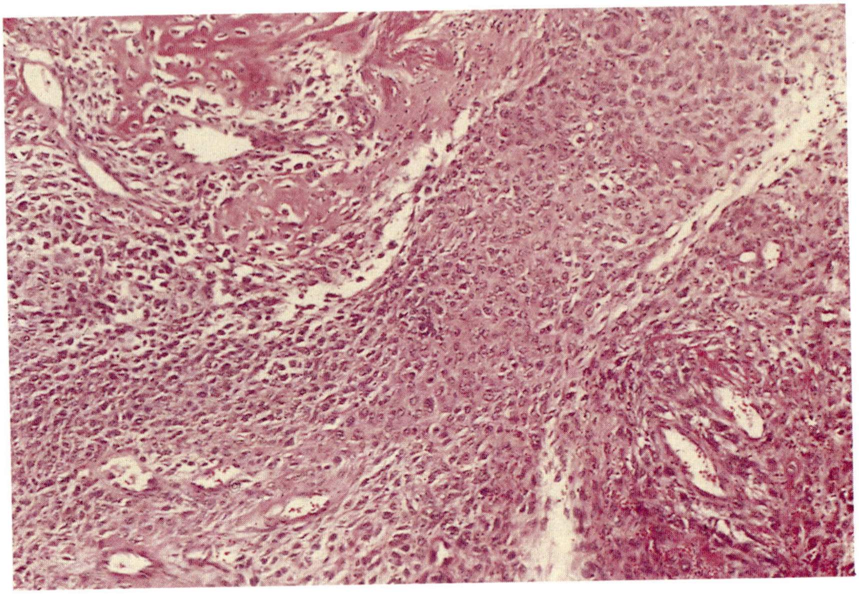

Fig. 17 - Osteosarcoma, osteoblastic. Malignant osteoblasts produce random foci of osteoid in a haphazard arrangement.

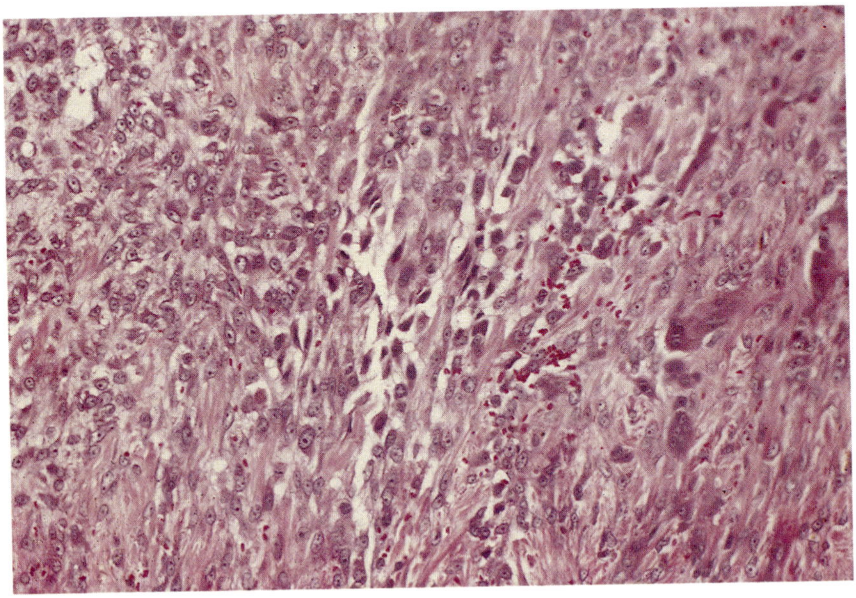

Fig. 18 - Osteosarcoma, osteoblastic, nonproductive. Although no osteosarcomas are completely devoid of osteoid, some produce very little.

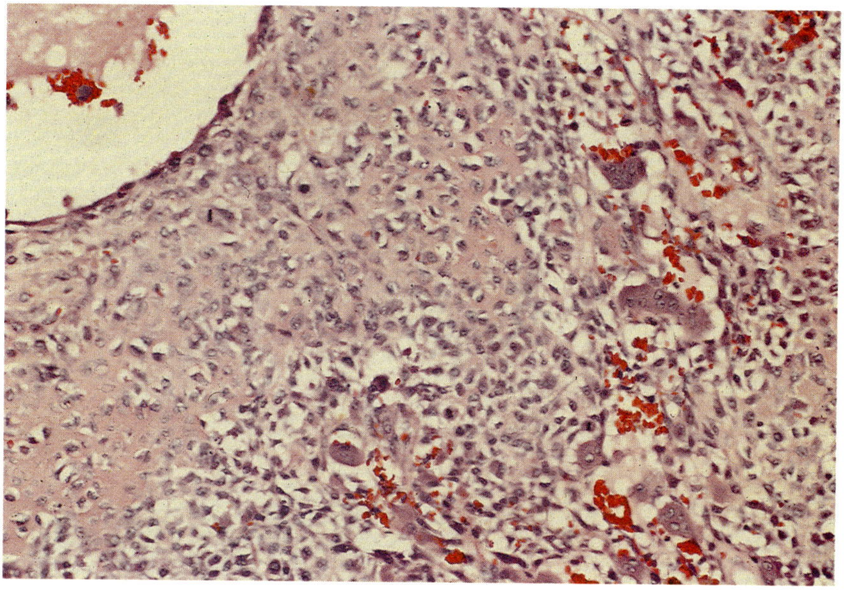

Fig. 19 - Osteosarcoma, osteoblastic, productive. Osteoid production is evident near a vascular space.

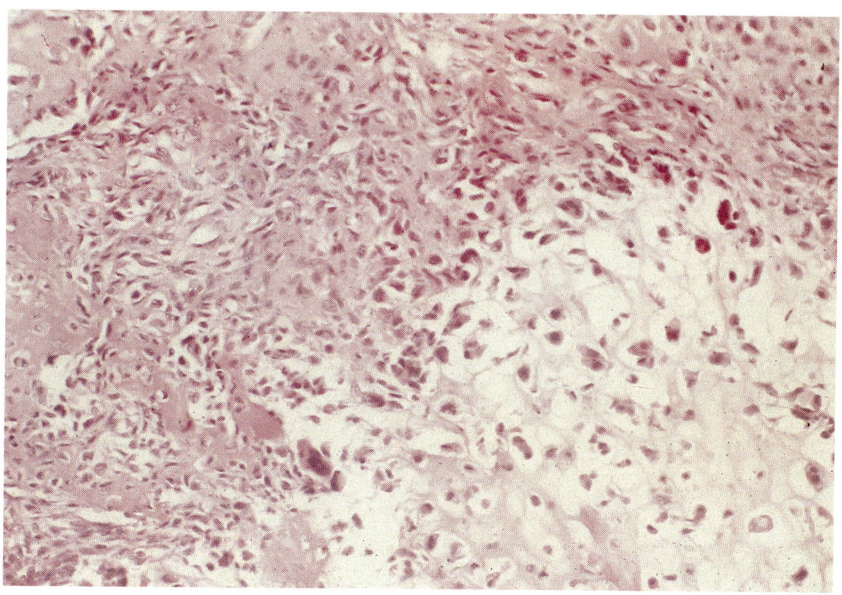

Fig. 20 - Osteosarcoma, chondroblastic. Although osteoid production identifies this tumor as osseous, islands of cartilage are a prominent feature.

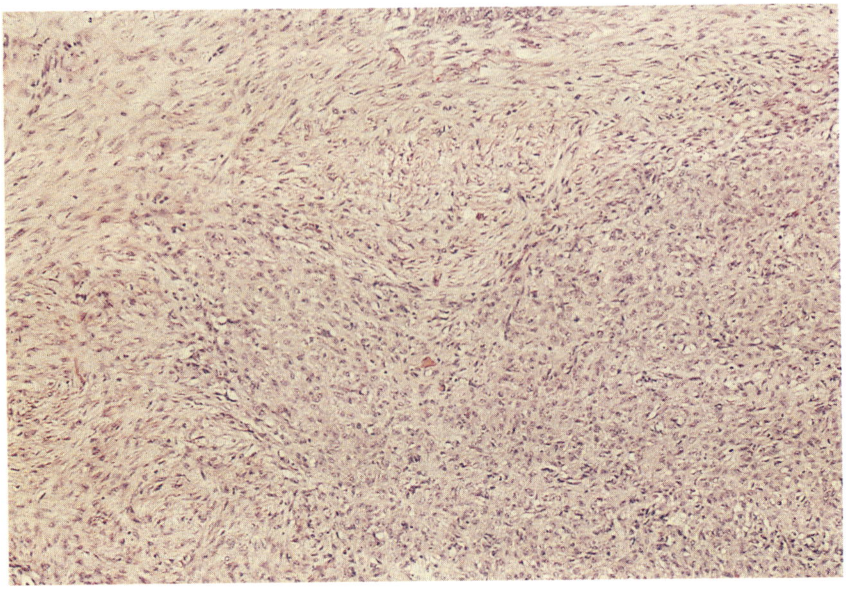

Fig. 21 - Osteosarcoma, fibroblastic. Malignant spindle-shaped osteoblasts.

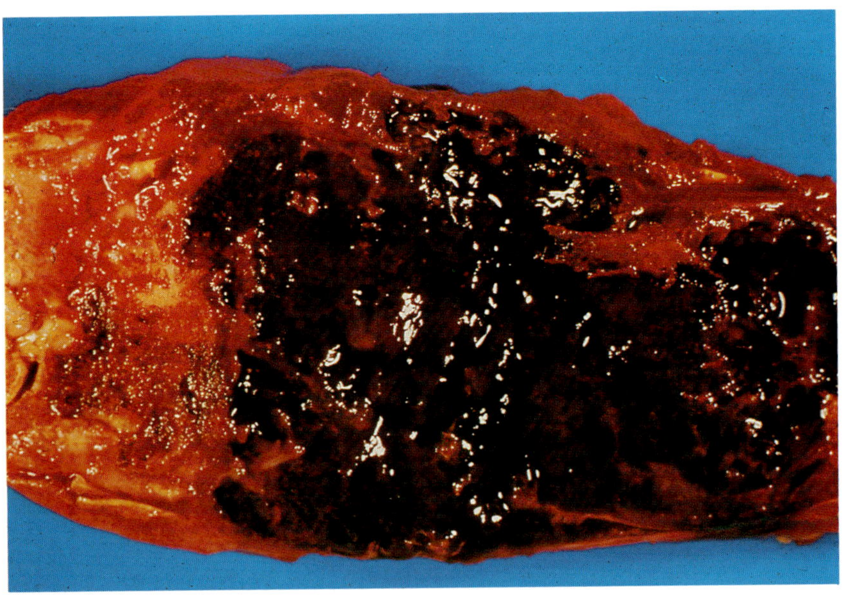

Fig. 22 - Osteosarcoma, telangiectatic, distal radius, dog, gross photo. Notice the replacement of medullary structures by bloody tumor tissue.

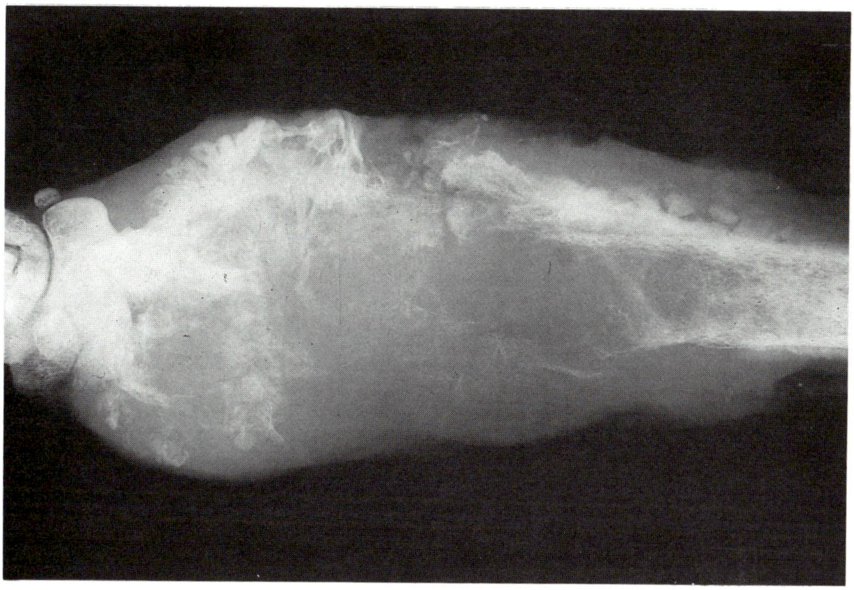

Fig. 23 - Osteosarcoma, telangiectactic. Specimen radiograph. Same as Figure 22. Notice nearly complete destruction of bone architecture and partial destruction of reactive bone on surface of dorsal cortex.

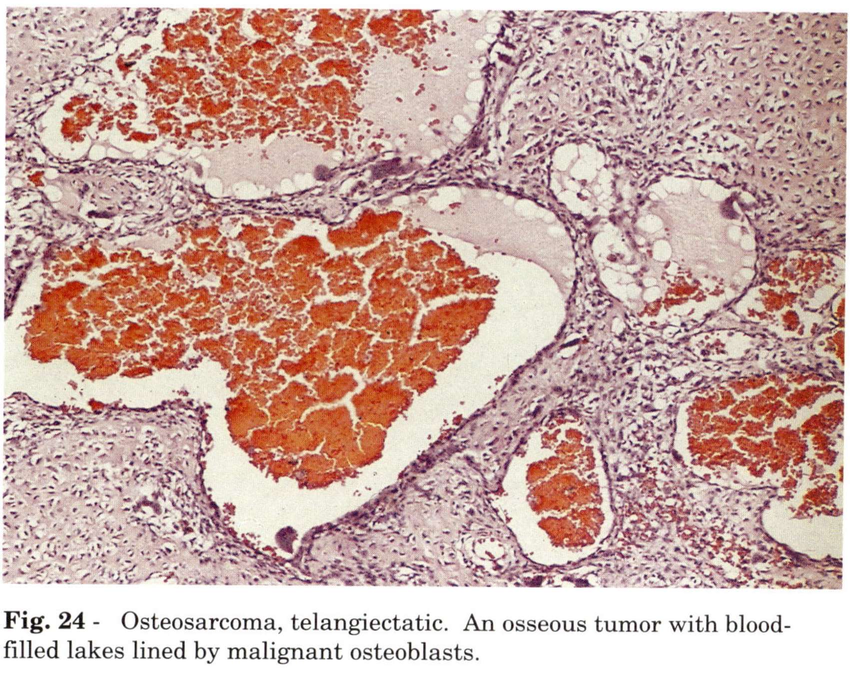

Fig. 24 - Osteosarcoma, telangiectatic. An osseous tumor with blood-filled lakes lined by malignant osteoblasts.

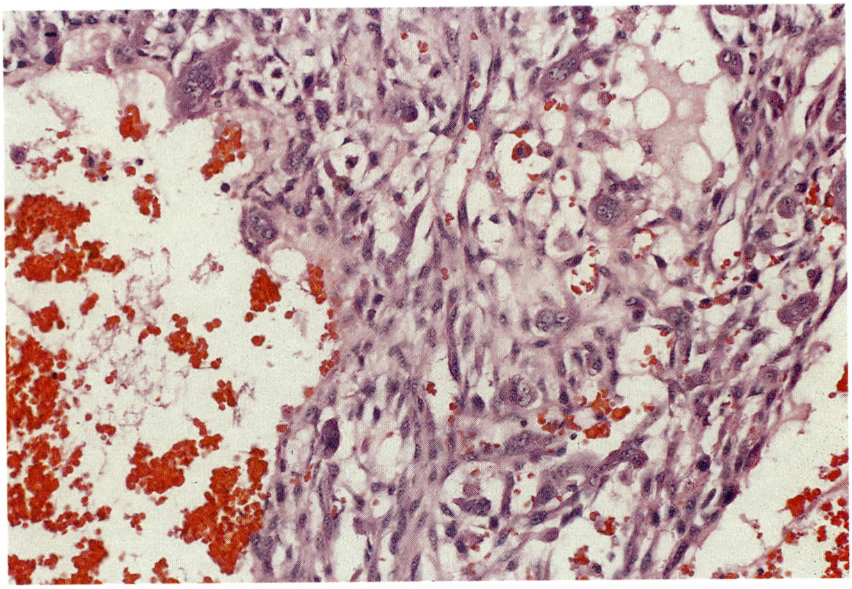

Fig. 25 - Osteosarcoma, telangiectatic. Higher magnification of Figure 24 showing absence of an endothelial lining of blood-filled cavities.

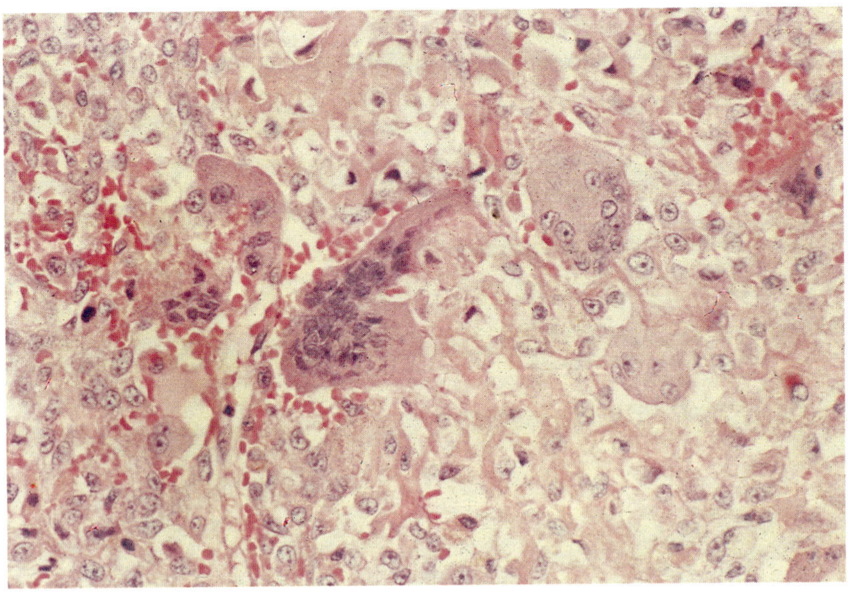

Fig. 26 - Osteosarcoma, giant cell type. This tumor is characterized by the fusion of numerous malignant osteoblasts to form tumor giant cells.

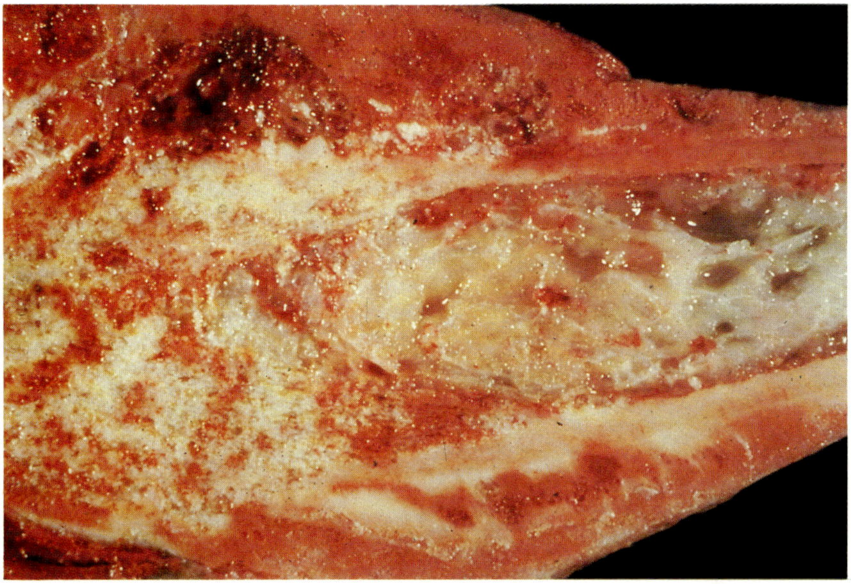

Fig. 27 - Chondrosarcoma. Gross photo. Islands of white glistening cartilage are present.

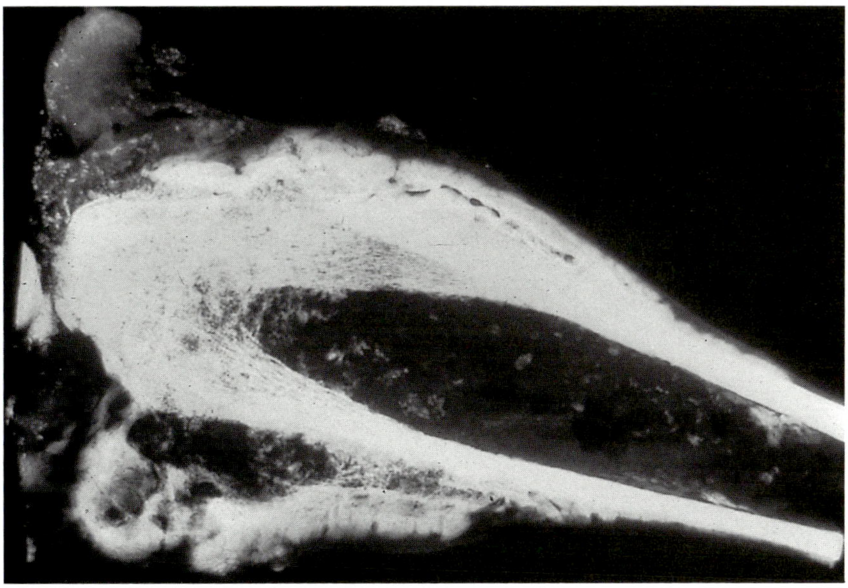

Fig. 28 - Chondrosarcoma. Slab radiograph. Proliferating cartilage produces a radiologic margin described as "Puffy," "Snowflake," or "Popcorn."

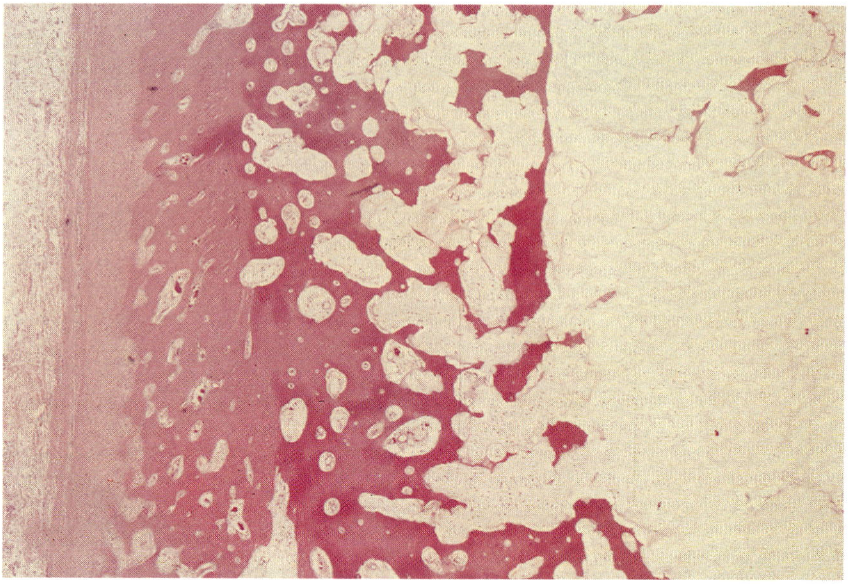

Fig. 29 - Chondrosarcoma. Invasion of preexisting bone by malignant chondroid elements.

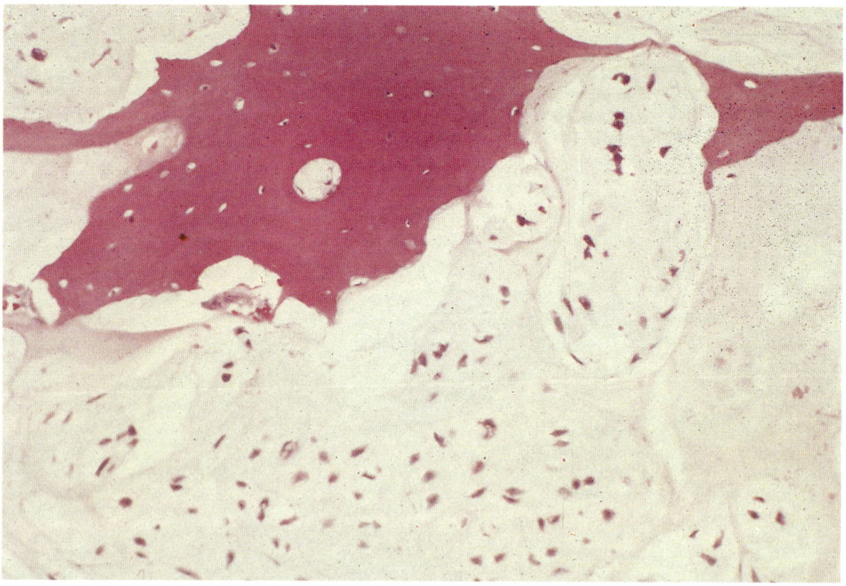

Fig. 30 - Chondrosarcoma. Higher magnification of Figure 29. Note the invasion of normal bone.

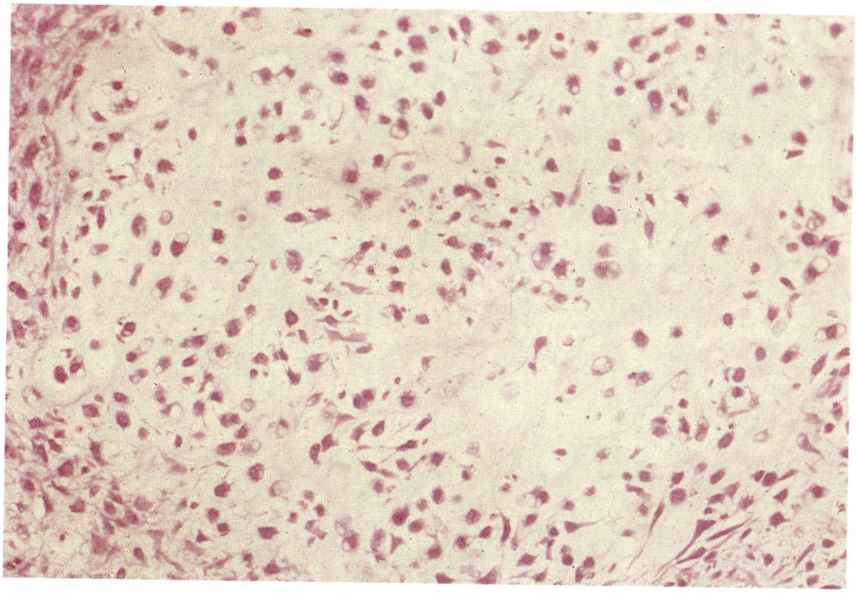

Fig. 31 - Chondrosarcoma. The pleomorphic cytology is prime evidence of malignancy.

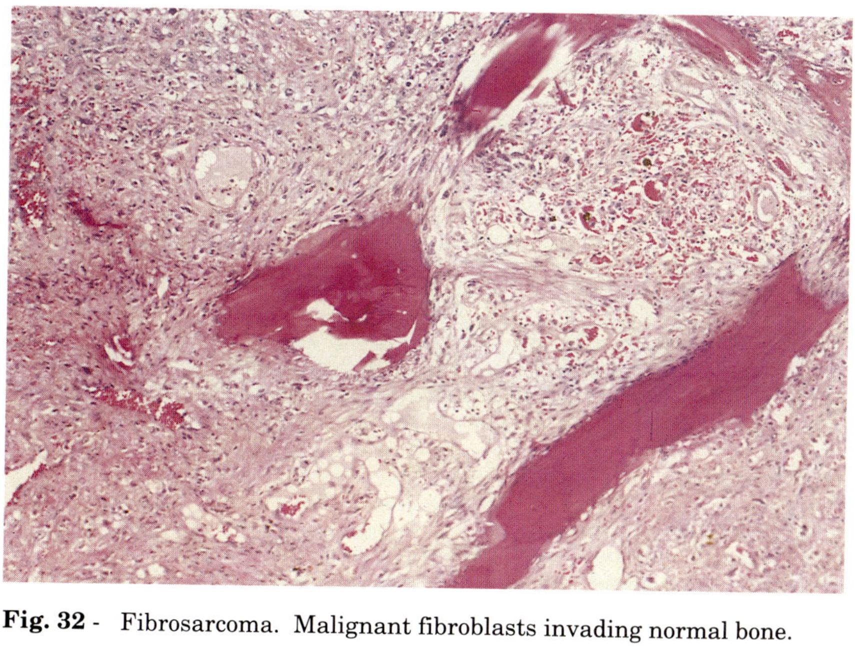

Fig. 32 - Fibrosarcoma. Malignant fibroblasts invading normal bone.

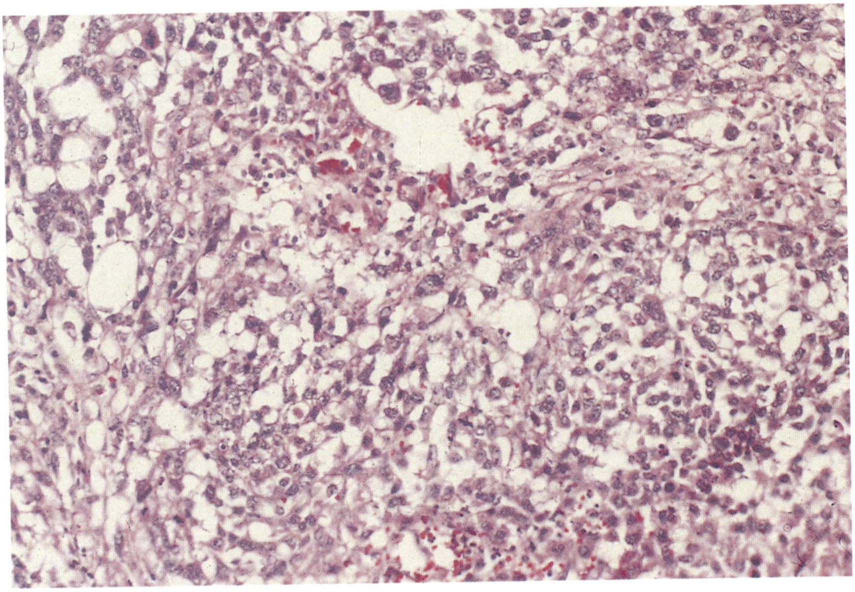

Fig. 33 - Fibrosarcoma. Anaplastic polygonal, stellate, and spindle-shaped cells make minimal collagen but no osteoid matrix.

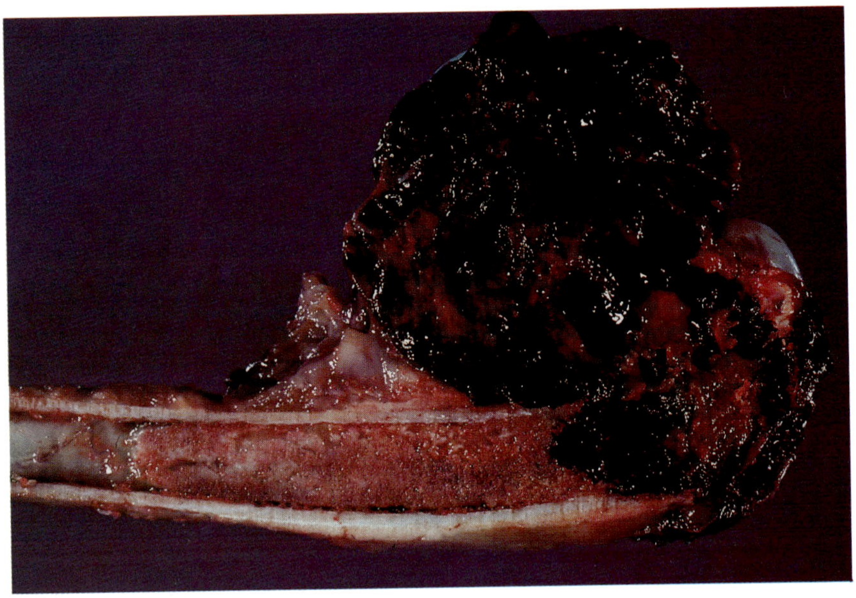

Fig. 34 - Hemangiosarcoma, distal femur, dog. Gross photo. Tumor has replaced distal metaphyseal spongiosa and compacta and extends into the soft tissues of the popliteal space.

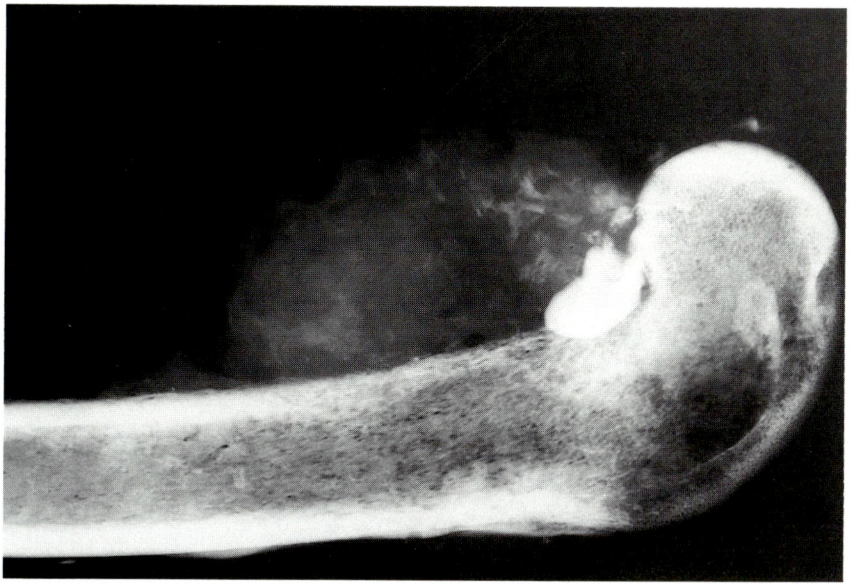

Fig. 35 - Hemangiosarcoma. Specimen radiograph of Figure 34. Note permeating pattern of bone destruction. Radiodensity in soft tissues is reactive bone from periosteum displaced by the tumor.

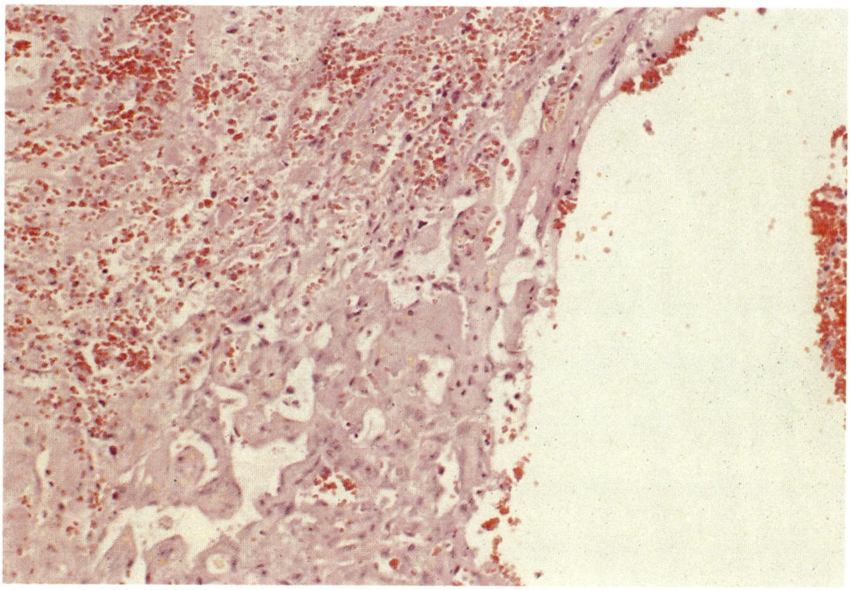

Fig. 36 - Hemangiosarcoma. As in the soft tissue variety, the tumor is composed of vascular spaces lined by malignant endothelium.

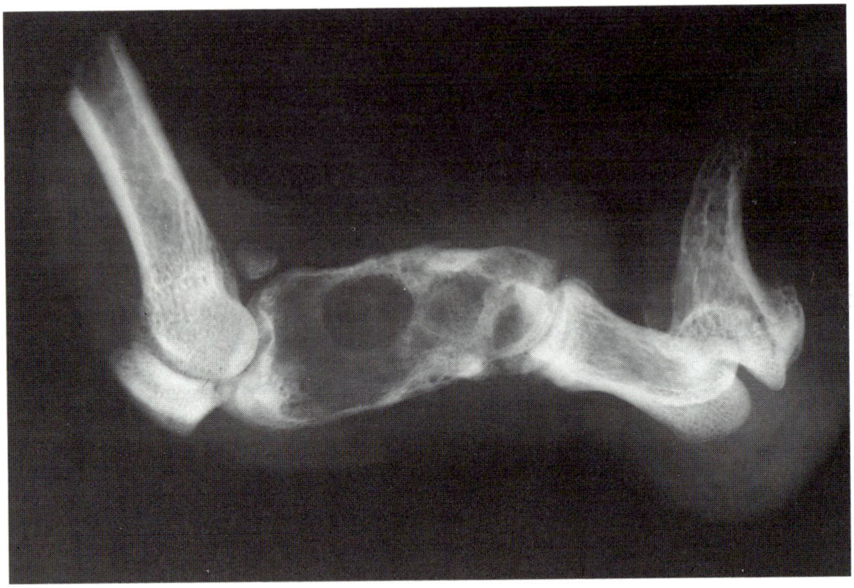

Fig. 37 - Giant cell tumor of bone, first phalanx. Radiograph. The lesion produced a discrete, expansile osteolytic lesion.

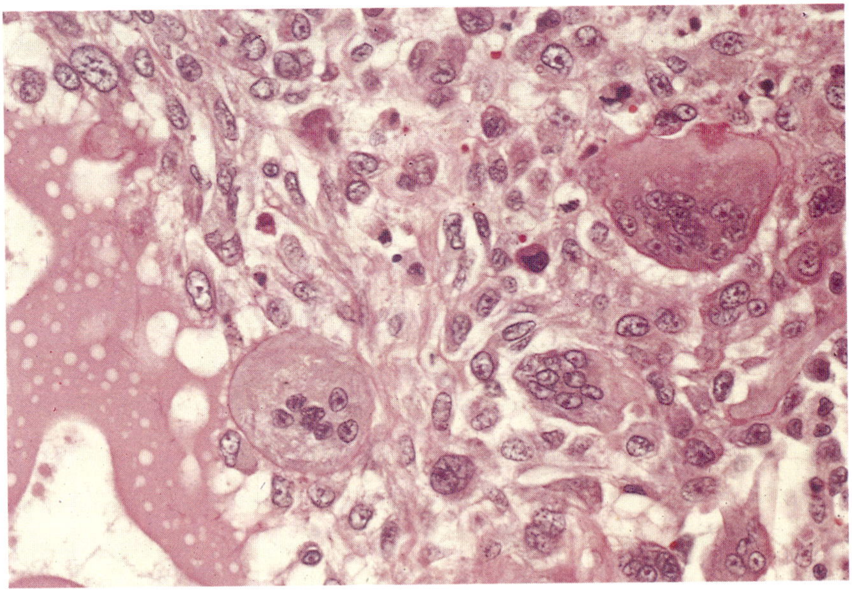

Fig. 38 - Giant cell tumor of bone. The nuclei all look similar, regardless if the cell is multinuclear or mononuclear. No osteoid is produced.

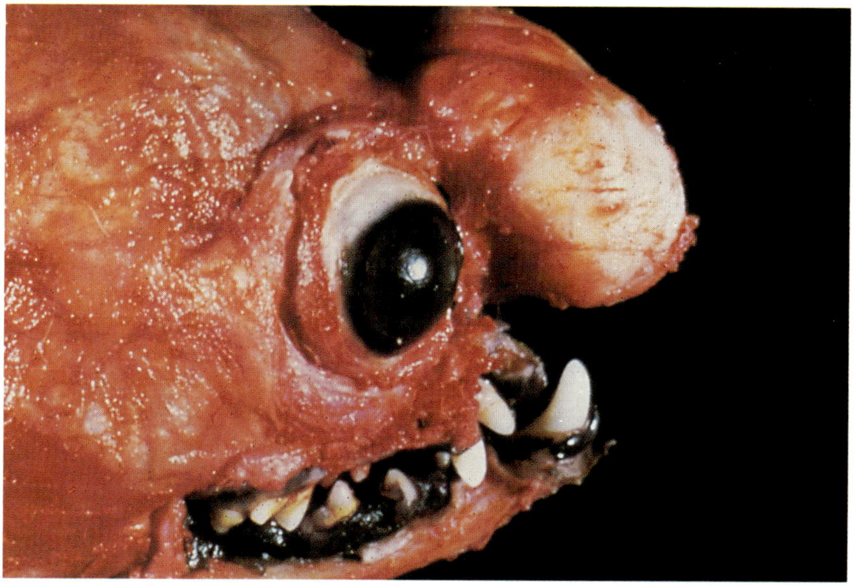

Fig. 39 - Multilobular tumor of bone, dog, skull. Gross appearance. The mass protrudes externally.

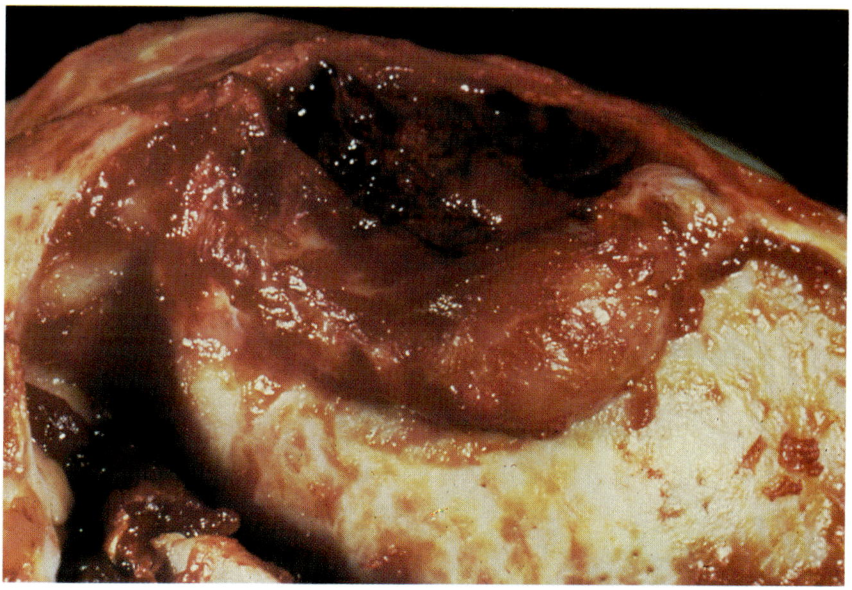

Fig. 40 - Multilobular tumor of bone, dog, skull. Intracranial gross appearance. The mass protrudes internally. The hematoma is incidental.

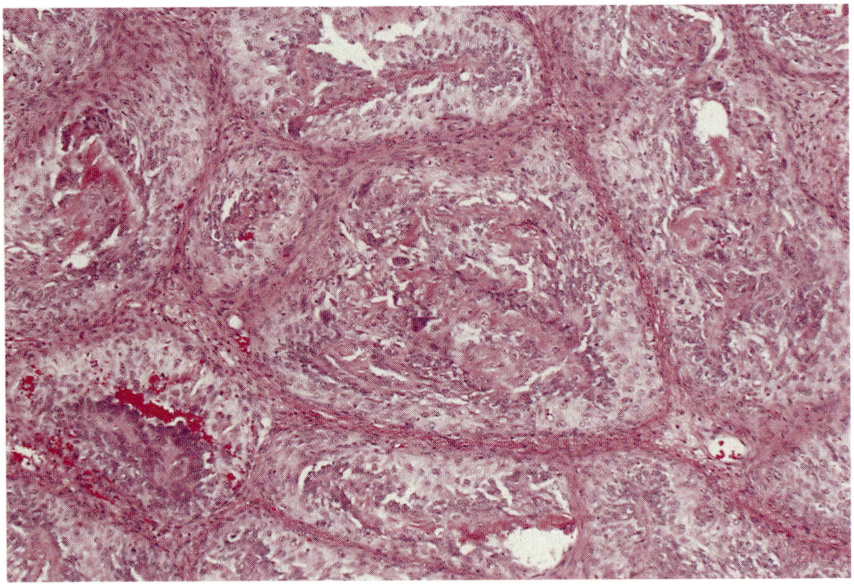

Fig. 41 - Multilobular tumor of bone. There are islands of bone and cartilage separated by septa of spindle cells.

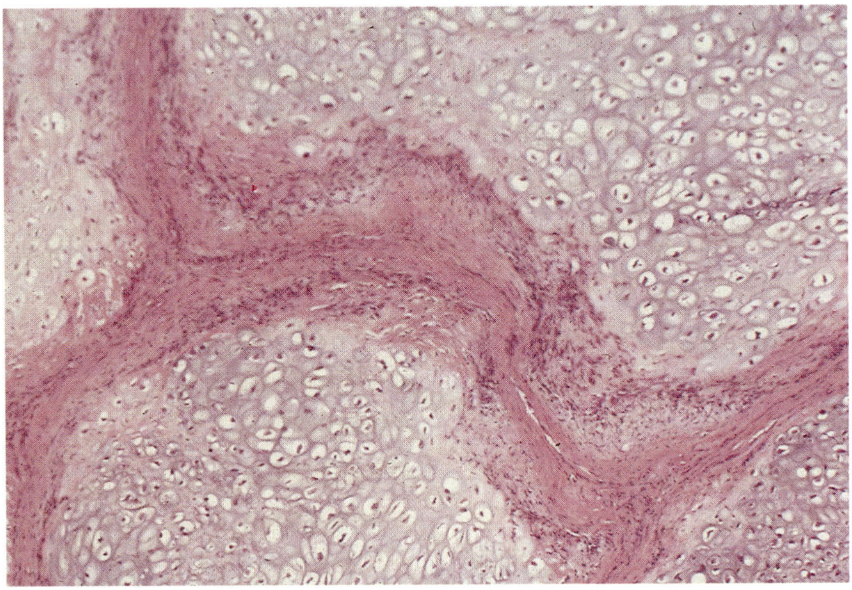

Fig. 42 - Multilobular tumor of bone. Lobules contain central islands of cartilage and bone matrix separated by thin fibrous septa containing spindle cells and small blood vessels.

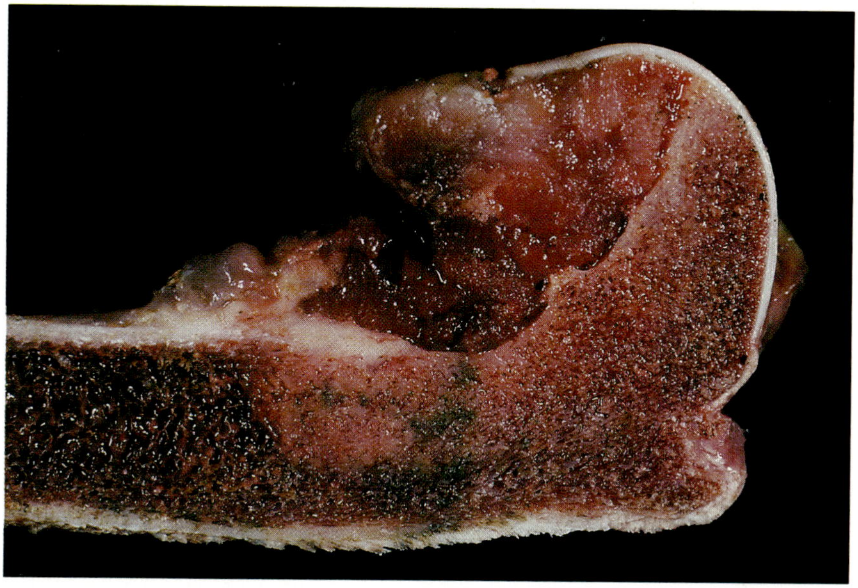

Fig. 43 - Periosteal chondrosarcoma, proximal humerus. Gross photo.

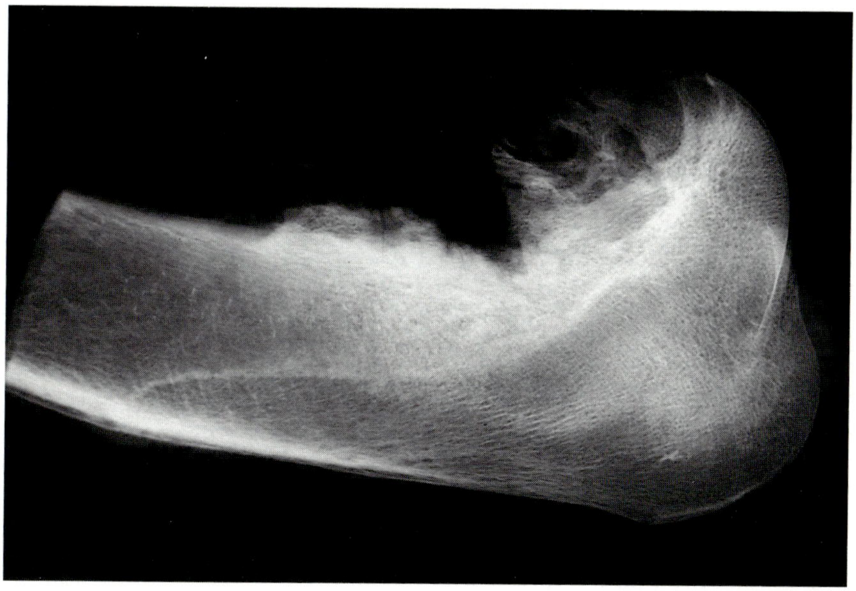

Fig. 44 - Periosteal chondrosarcoma. Specimen radiograph. Same animal as Figure 43. Note increased bone density along the base of the tumor, indicating its low aggressive behavior.

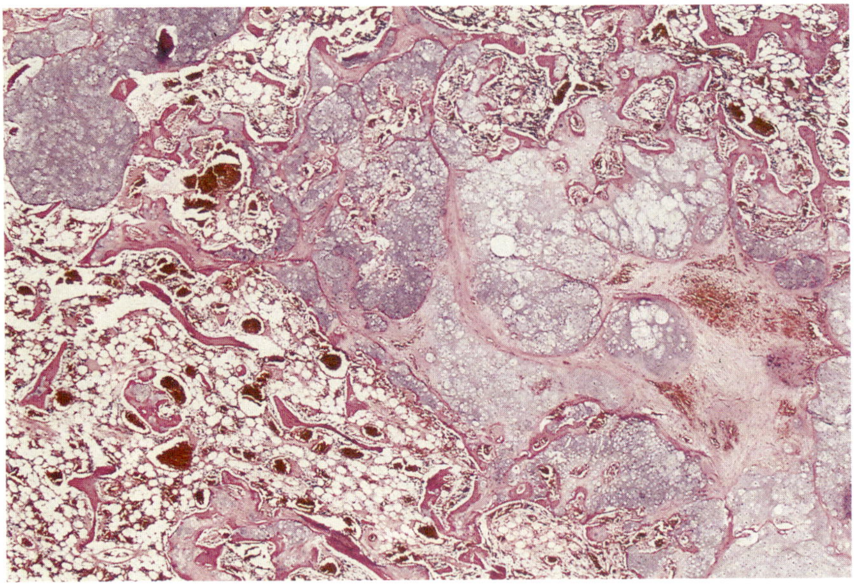

Fig. 45 - Periosteal chondrosarcoma. Histological appearance.

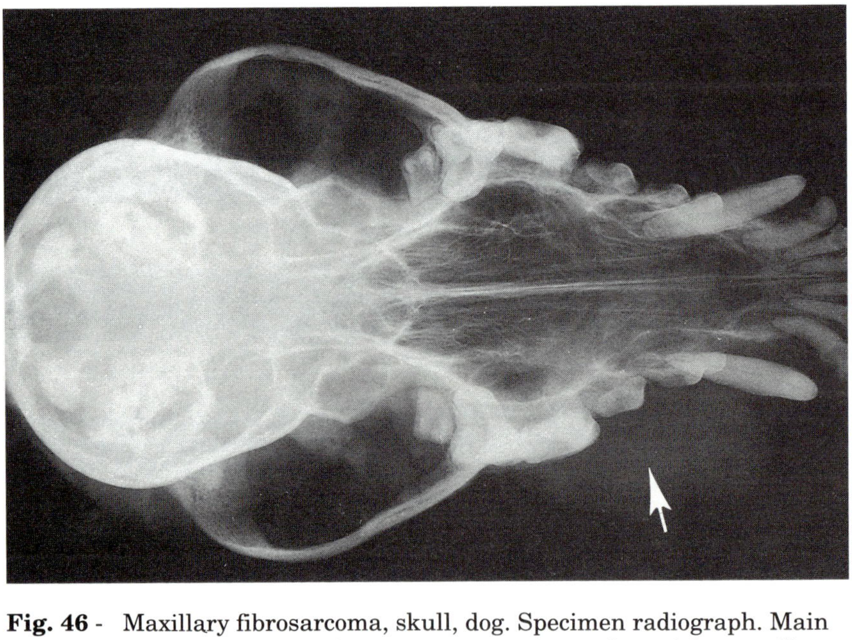

Fig. 46 - Maxillary fibrosarcoma, skull, dog. Specimen radiograph. Main radiographic finding is the soft tissue mass on the surface of the maxilla (arrow).

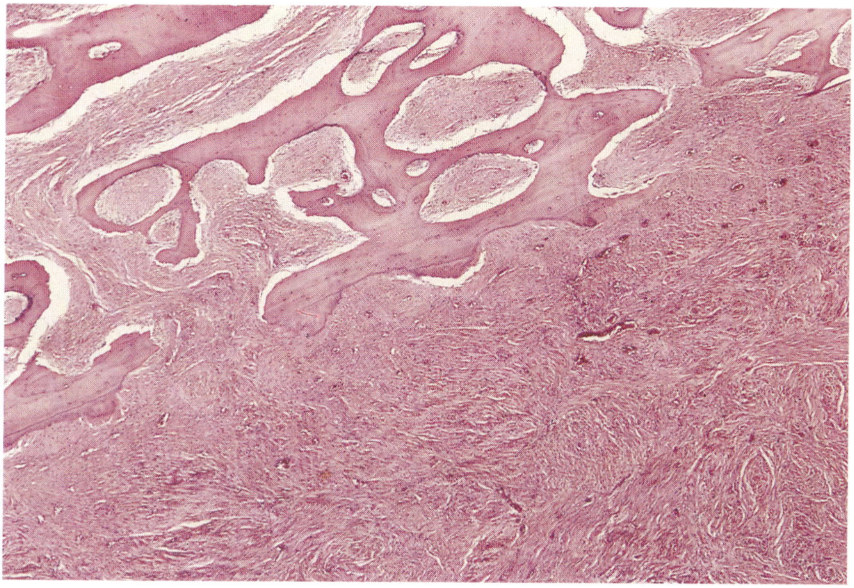

Fig. 47 - Maxillary fibrosarcoma, head, dog. Histologic appearance. Tumor destroys and invades underlying cortical bone of maxilla.

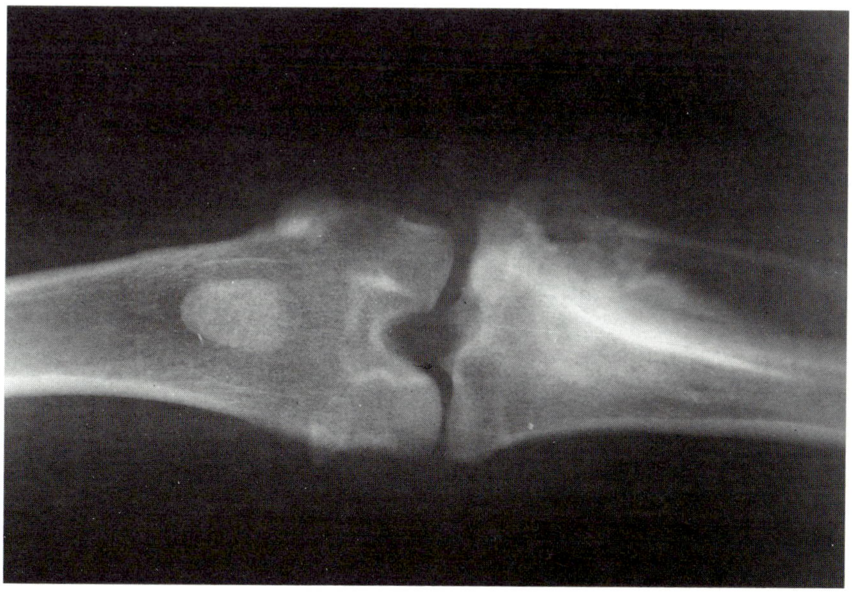

Fig. 48 - Periosteal osteosarcoma. Clinical radiograph, proximal tibia, dog. Productive bony tumor arises from the surface of the lateral cortex.

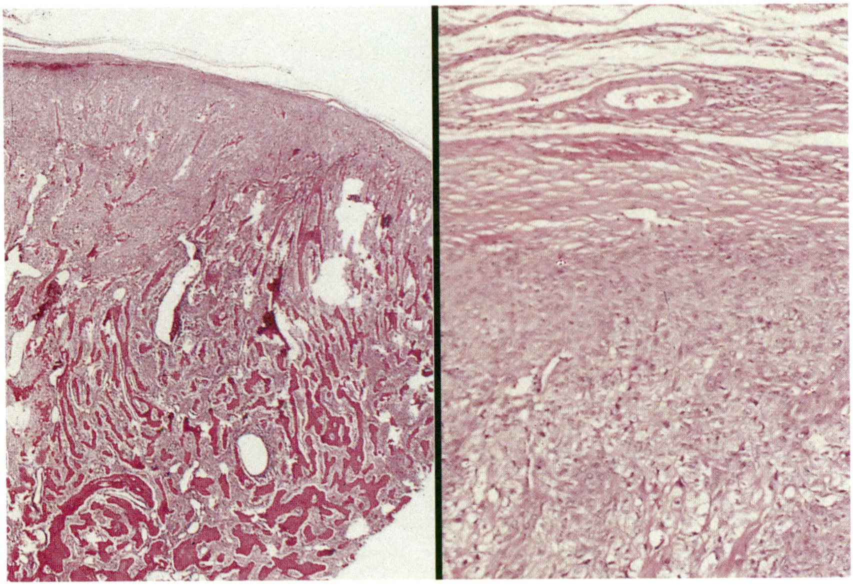

Fig. 49 A & B - Periosteal osteosarcoma. Same case as Figure 48. A) Well-differentiated histologic appearance. B) Higher magnification.

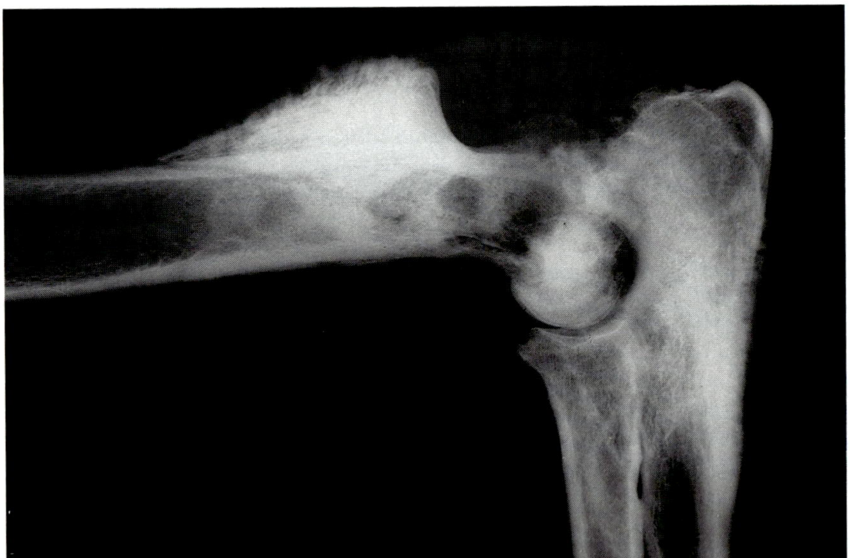

Fig. 50 - Synovial sarcoma. Specimen radiograph, elbow, dog. A soft tissue mass is centered on the elbow. Bone destruction is present in the joint capsule insertion lines. Periosteal reaction borders the soft tissue mass.

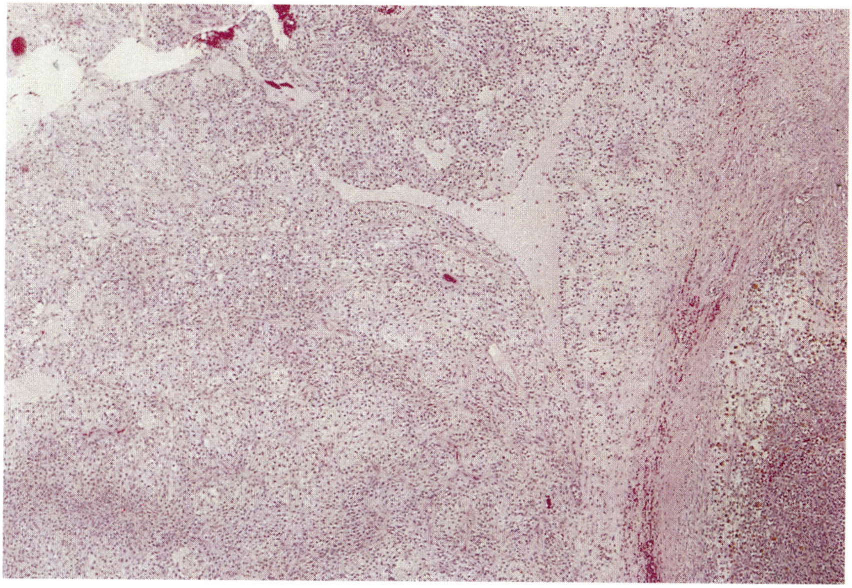

Fig. 51 - Synovial sarcoma, dog, elbow joint. Histologic appearance, low magnification.

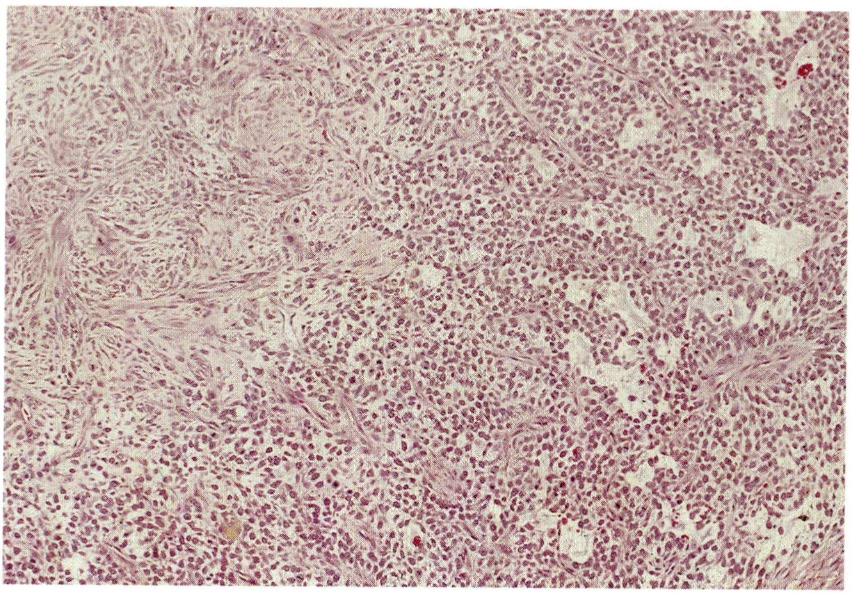

Fig. 52 - Synovial sarcoma, same as Figure 51, higher magnification. Epithelioid cells predominate over spindle cells. Numerous cavities are present, lined by synovioblasts and filled with connective tissue mucin.

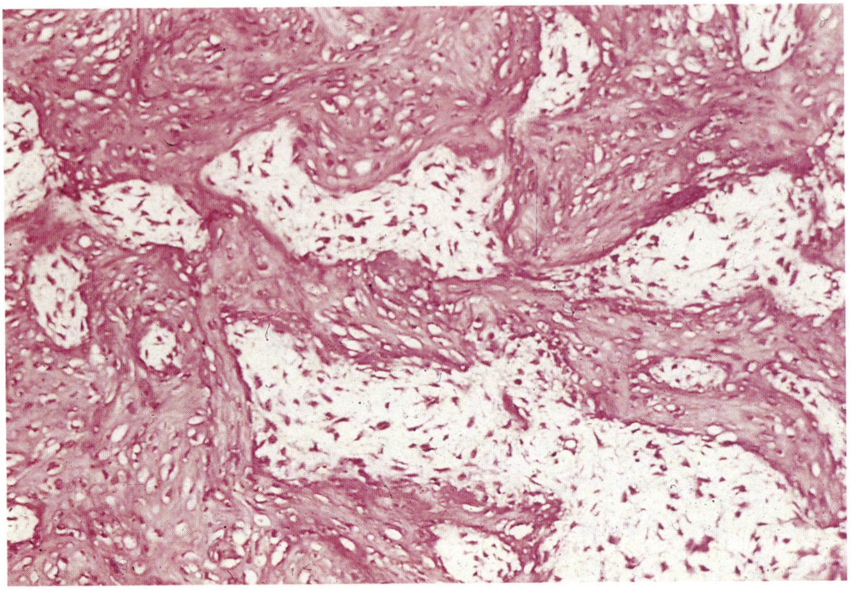

Fig. 53 - Fibrous dysplasia, cat. “Naked” spicules of bone, having no lining osteoblasts, are separated by loose fibrous connective tissue.

Subject Index

NOTES

NOTES

NOTES

NOTES